SUMMER MASTITIS

Current Topics in Veterinary Medicine and Animal Science

Recent publications

1984

26. Manipulation of Growth in Farm Animals, edited by J.F. Roche and D. O'Callaghan. ISBN 0-89838-617-8
27. Latent Herpes Virus Infections in Veterinary Medicine, edited by G. Wittmann, R.M. Gaskell and H.-J. Rziha. ISBN 0-89838-622-5
28. Grassland Beef Production, edited by W. Holmes. ISBN 0-89838-650-0
29. Recent Advances in Virus Diagnosis, edited by M.S. McNulty and J.B. McFerran. ISBN 0-89838-674-8
30. The Male in Farm Animal Reproduction, edited by M. Courot. ISBN 0-89838-682-9

1985

31. Endocrine Causes of Seasonal and Lactational Anestrus in Farm Animals, edited by F. Ellendorff and F. Elsaesser. ISBN 0-89838-738-8
32. Brucella Melitensis, edited by J.M. Verger and M. Plommet. ISBN 0-89838-742-6

1986

33. Diagnosis of Mycotoxicoses, edited by J.L. Richard and J.R. Thurston. ISBN 0-89838-751-5
34. Embryonic Mortality in Farm Animals, edited by J.M. Sreenan and M.G. Diskin. ISBN 0-89838-772-8
35. Social Space for Domestic Animals, edited by R. Zayan. ISBN 0-89838-773-6
36. The Present State of Leptospirosis Diagnosis and Control, edited by W.A. Ellis and T.W.A. Little. ISBN 0-89838-777-9
37. Acute Virus Infections of Poultry, edited by J.B. McFerran and M.S. McNulty. ISBN 0-89838-809-0

1987

38. Evaluation and Control of Meat Quality in Pigs, edited by P.V. Tarrant, G. Eikelenboom and G. Monin. ISBN 0-89838-854-6
39. Follicular Growth and Ovulation Rate in Farm Animals, edited by J.F. Roche and D. O'Callaghan. ISBN 0-89838-855-4
40. Cattle Housing Systems, Lameness and Behaviour, edited by H.K. Wierenga and D.J. Peterse. ISBN 0-89838-862-7
41. Physiological and Pharmacological Aspects of the Reticulo-rumen, edited by L.A.A. Ooms, A.D. Degryse and A.S.J.P.A.M. van Miert. ISBN 0-89838-878-3
42. Biology of Stress in Farm Animals: An Integrative Approach, edited by P.R. Wiepkema and P.W.M. van Adrichem. ISBN 0-89838-895-3
43. Helminth Zoonoses, edited by S. Geerts, V. Kumar and J. Brandt. ISBN 0-89838-896-1
44. Energy Metabolism in Farm Animals: Effects of Housing, Stress and Disease, edited by M.W.A. Verstegen and A.M. Henken. ISBN 0-89838-974-7
45. Summer Mastitis, edited by G. Thomas, H.J. Over, U. Vecht and P. Nansen. ISBN 0-89838-982-8

Summer Mastitis

A Workshop in the Community Programme
for the Coordination of Agricultural Research,
held at the Central Veterinary Institute,
Lelystad, The Netherlands, 23–24 October 1986

Sponsored by the Commission of the European Communities,
Directorate General for Agriculture, Coordination of Agricultural Research

Edited by

G. THOMAS & H.J. OVER

Department of Parasitology, Central Veterinary Institute
Lelystad, The Netherlands

U. VECHT

Department of Bacteriology, Central Veterinary Institute
Lelystad, The Netherlands

P. NANSEN

Institute of Hygiene and Microbiology,
Royal Veterinary and Agricultural University,
Copenhagen, Denmark

1987

MARTINUS NIJHOFF PUBLISHERS
A MEMBER OF THE KLUWER ACADEMIC PUBLISHERS GROUP
DORDRECHT – BOSTON – LANCASTER
FOR THE COMMISSION OF THE EUROPEAN COMMUNITIES

Distributors

for the United States and Canada: Kluwer Academic Publishers, P.O. Box 358, Accord Station, Hingham, MA 02018-0358, USA
for the UK and Ireland: Kluwer Academic Publishers, MTP Press Limited, Falcon House, Queen Square, Lancaster LA1 1RN, UK
for all other countries: Kluwer Academic Publishers Group, Distribution Center, P.O. Box 322, 3300 AH Dordrecht, The Netherlands

Library of Congress Cataloging in Publication Data

Summer mastitis.

    (Current topics in veterinary medicine and animal
science)
    Includes bibliographies.
    1. Summer mastitis--Congresses. I. Thomas, G.
II. Commission of the European Communities.
Coordination of Agricultural Research. III. Series.
SF967.M3S86 1987   636.2'089819   87-26669

ISBN-13:978-94-010-8015-6   e-ISBN-13:978-94-009-3373-6
DOI: 10.1007/978-94-009-3373-6

EUR 10819 EN

Book information

Publication arranged by Commission of the European Communities, Directorate-General Telecommunications, Information Industries and Innovation.

Copyright / legal notice

TABLE OF CONTENTS

PREFACE

PREFACE

This Community meeting has been organised, since over the past 15 years in different countries of Western Europe including Scandinavia, a lot of research has been directed to the summer mastitis problem.

Summer mastitis in cattle is a well known disease which, because of its abruptness and the difficulties concerned in defining the predisposing factors and the pathogens involved, is hard to control. Moreover, as it is anticipated that in the transmission of the bacteria one or more dipterans are involved, the complexity in defining the disease and hence co-ordinating our scientific knowledge in relation to practical control was stimulus enough for this workshop to be organised.

Our aims can be summarised in the following goals:

1. Exchange of information in the practical, technical and scientific field in order to stimulate a co-ordinated research approach at a time in which the cattle husbandry sector is under great economical stress.
2. Inform research workers from countries where the disease is or seems to be, not endemic, on aspects that might be of interest for them in the approach of comparable problems.
3. To draw up conclusions and recommendations with regard to future research activities in order to avoid needless duplication of effort.

With these goals in mind the organising committee has set up this programme as a forum for activities and to synthesise and compile the results of the research activities in a single comprehensive publication. We would also like to take this opportunity to express our thanks to the Directorate-General for Agriculture of the Commission of the European Communities. Moreover, thanks are due to numerous anonymous collaborators who functioned in a supporting role and helped to make the workshop a success, in particular Mrs C.D. Propsma-van der Haven whose invaluable assistance in preparing the manuscript is gratefully acknowledged.

H.J. Over
P. Nansen
G. Thomas
U. Vecht

Lelystad and Copenhagen, December 1986.

1. EPIDEMIOLOGY OF SUMMER MASTITIS

Chairmen J.E. Hillerton & H.J. Over

THE EPIDEMIOLOGY OF SUMMER MASTITIS

J.E. Hillerton

Milking and Mastitis Centre,
AFRC Institute for Research on Animal Diseases,
Compton, Berks, RG16 0NN, U.K.

ABSTRACT

The incidence of summer mastitis, or more accurately *A. pyogenes*/anaerobe mastitis, is considered in terms of animals at risk, stage of gestation, season of the year and geographical occurrence of the infection. It is significant that a large proportion of cases occur in the spring in housed animals. However the majority of cases are associated with autumn calving cows and heifers, at summer pasture.

Susceptibility to infection varies with the age of the cow, breed, breeding and husbandry. Disease is coincident with the occurrence of a potential vector, the fly *Hydrotaea irritans*, in summer but not in winter/spring. The mechanism of infection might be similar in both seasons once the cow is contaminated by the bacteria. The absence of the vector in spring may explain the much lower incidence of disease then.

Little is known of the effects of husbandry, especially nutritional and environmental stresses, on increasing susceptibility to infection. This should be remedied. More accurate diagnosis is required, it is at best 80% accurate, to confirm *A. pyogenes*/anaerobe mastitis, as anaerobic culturing is rarely used routinely.

INTRODUCTION

Summer mastitis is one colloquiallism for an imprecisely defined infection. It can be assumed to include all clinical infections of the non-lactating mammary gland of cattle from which a complex bacterial flora is isolated. The bacterial pathogens should include *Actinomyces pyogenes* and anaerobic bacteria or evidence that such a mixture has been involved in the infection. The disease is recognised as occurring in an epidemic form in the developed dairy industries of northern Europe and Japan. It is most prevalent in the summer. This is believed to be related to the high number of animals at risk and the occurrence of a fly vector encouraging rapid spread of infection at this time.

The fine details from all reports in the literature have recently been compiled by Tolle *et al.* (1985) and will not be repeated here, instead some of the evidence surrounding the dogma of summer mastitis will be examined. Using data mostly from England and Wales, the following will be considered; the incidence of the disease in relation to geography, annual and seasonal patterns, animals at risk; susceptibility, especially related to breed, physiology and population; and coincidences such as other infections, flies and animal husbandry.

INCIDENCE

There is a plethora of incidence data complicated by different breeds of cattle from different areas and collected in different years. A consensus would indicate that 20—60% of dairy herds in U.K., Eire, the Netherlands, Belgium, Luxembourg, West Germany, East Germany, Denmark, Sweden, Finland, Poland and the Baltic states are infected annually with one or more cases. The incidence figures vary from year to year but generally the same herds always suffer from summer mastitis. It would appear that the incidence of disease has decreased considerably in recent years especially in the Netherlands (Sol et al., 1985). There is some evidence from England and Wales (Table 1) that fewer herds have been affected recently and with fewer cases per herd. However, whether this reduction is real and related to control measures is unproven as the results show that the level has only dropped to that prevalent when the survey commenced 8 years ago. The early 1980's were marked by a higher incidence of summer mastitis.

The same annual pattern does not feature over the whole of northern Europe, possibly because of differences in weather, although the patterns for West Germany and England and Wales appear similar (Tolle and Reichmuth, 1985).

Incidence data are usually based on clinical cases and figures can be separated for dry cows, pregnant heifers and non-pregnant heifers. These show that a similar incidence occurs in dry cows and pregnant heifers, 1—3% of animals at risk, with usually more pregnant heifers affected. Non-pregnant animals suffer a much lower incidence, 0.2—0.5% animals at risk (Tolle et al., 1985 and Table 1).

TABLE 1.   Incidence of summer mastitis as determined on farms by the Milk Marketing Board of England and Wales (O'Rourke, et al., 1984; O'Rourke, pers. comm.).

Year	No. of herds	% infected herds	No. cases/ herd	% animals infected		
				dry cows	pregnant heifers	non-pregnant heifers
1978	248	43	3.5	—	—	—
1979	393	40	2.4	—	—	—
1980	416	43	2.6	—	—	—
1981	391	59	4.1	—	—	—
1982	499	54	2.6	—	—	—
1983	484	42	2.7	1.2	1.9	0.6
1984	251	40	2.5	1.2	1.1	0.4
1985	275	35	2.1	1.0	1.5	0.5

The use of dry cow therapy is widespread throughout northern Europe. Whereas, before the advent of such treatment most dry period infections occurred soon after drying off, the risk has now shifted, to the latter half of the dry period (Hillerton *et al.*, 1987). Fewer animals are therefore effectively at risk until the prophylactic effect of dry cow therapy has declined. On this basis the true incidence in dry cows could be up to double the quoted figures, despite fewer animals in total being infected.

It is often assumed that because an infection is labelled summer mastitis it is an *A. pyogenes*/anaerobe infection. The accuracy of diagnosis will affect the incidence figures. Of 252 summer mastitis cases in England and Wales examined in 1983 and 1984, 80% were proven by bacteriology to have been correctly diagnosed as *A. pyogenes*/anaerobe infections (Hillerton *et al.*, 1987). The incidence data quoted from this study are based on these cases and therefore are true incidence rates.

Summer mastitis is considered most prevalent in autumn calving herds where most animals are at risk in the peak months of incidence, July, August and September. Spring calving herds also experience the problem (Meaney and Egan, 1982). Mastitis, from which *A. pyogenes* is isolated, occurs throughout the year but in most instances no anaerobic culture is attempted. Bearing this restriction in mind the U.K. Veterinary Investigation Service figures provide an approximate monthly incidence of *A. pyogenes* mastitis in cases reported for investigation. It is not known if all cases are in non-lactating animals but most are assumed to be as the usual incidence of *A. pyogenes* mastitis in lactating cows is < 0.7 cases/week/1000 cows (unpublished field data).

The results (Fig 1) suggest that most cases occur in August as expected and this is certainly a gross underestimate of the true picture as few veterinarians will bother to send for further investigation samples from a dry cow mastitis at this time of year. However using National Milk Records data from 1600 herds (S.V. Morant, pers. comm.) to weight the cases by the number of animals at risk, there is an obvious spring peak in incidence of *A. pyogenes* mastitis. Similar results are known from England in 1967–1970 (unpublished field data), a cohort of 273 herds closely monitored in England in 1980–1982 (Francis *et al.*, 1986) and from Schleswig–Holstein in 1950–1964 (Untermann, 1965). In all these surveys when corrected for animals at risk, the spring peak was equal to, or greater than, the autumn peak.

Local variations in the disease incidence are numerous and poorly explained. There is evidence that incidence is higher on well drained sandy soils (Saes, 1970). Investigation of this in England has not confirmed the observation but this may be due to the relative absence of dairying from sandy soils in England. These sandy soils are mostly acidic heathland unlike the soils of Limburg and Schleswig–Holstein. Correlation of dairying and summer mastitis with soil type in England and Wales is not with sandy soils but with soils with a high organic matter content which is similar to the soils of Limburg and Schleswig–Holstein. Although not necessarily well draining, these soils have an open structure and so can be construed as particularly suitable to support active fly larvae.

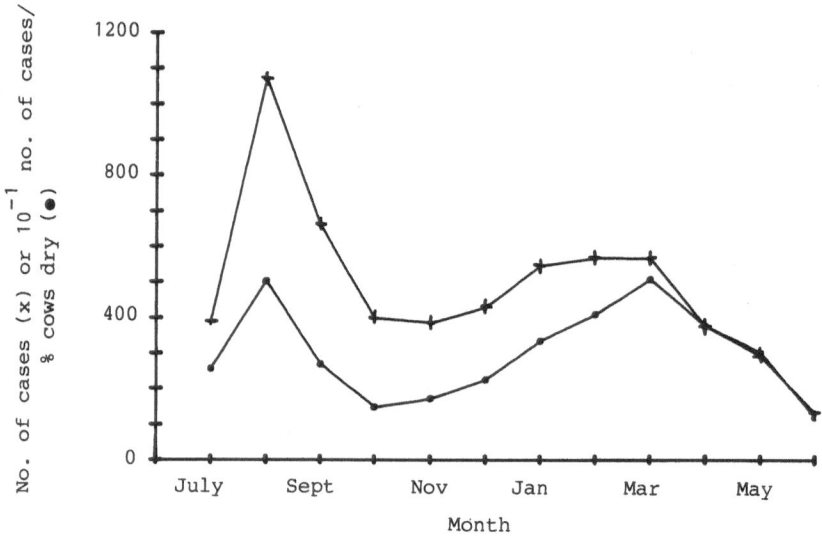

Figure 1. + — monthly incidence of *A. pyogenes* mastitis as reported to the U.K. Veterinary Investigation Service, total numbers reported from 1978–1985.
● — monthly incidence of *A. pyogenes* mastitis, reported as above, weighted by the proportion of dairy cows dry in that month. (MAFF, 1975–1985).

Little is known of the incidence in beef herds where cows are dry for a much longer period, but the disease occurs in Charolais cattle in France and in mixed breed suckler herds in Scotland where the local incidence, up to 20%, is often higher than in dairy animals (15%) (R. Plenderleith, pers. comm.).

SUSCEPTIBILITY

Overall, the incidence of *A. pyogenes*/anaerobe mastitis is 10 fold higher in dry cows than in lactating cows. This may be related to the relative composition of milk and dry secretion. *A. pyogenes* grows poorly at pH 6.6, as found in milk, but well in alkaline media, as in dry secretion (Hillerton, unpublished). It is a relatively slow growing organism which establishes with difficulty in the lactating gland. When infection is found in housed, lactating cows it is probably related to high environmental challenge from other sites of infection (*e.g.* genital tract), lesions and a poorly maintained milking machine.

The incidence of summer mastitis in Friesian cattle is much higher than in other breeds. In Schleswig–Holstein the incidence in Friesians is 3 times that in the Angler (Sieck, 1982). Breed differences also appear likely in Denmark, the Netherlands and the U.K. with Friesians being most susceptible. In East Germany breeding experiments indicated that the susceptibility was much lower in Jersey/Friesian crosses than in pure-bred Friesians (Muller, 1977).

Within breeds there are noticeable differences in susceptibility to infection. In Denmark the sire has been shown to influence susceptibility (Hansen and Nielsen, 1983) and sire is known to affect overall susceptibility to mastitis as well as other mucosal infections (Lie, 1985). Evidence is now being gathered that effects of the dam are also distinguishable (A.M. Russell, pers. comm.). The different susceptibilities are partly related to milk yield and rate of milking suggesting that the diameter of the teat duct and its closing ability are related to bacterial invasion of the udder. Also teat size and colour might influence attractiveness to vectors. Breeds with small teats and hairy udders seem to contract summer mastitis less frequently.

The effect of pregnancy on disease susceptibility is marked. Pregnant heifers are 10 fold more susceptible than non-pregnant heifers or calves and susceptibility appears higher in late gestation animals. Whilst this is true for dry cows this is biased since cows are rarely dry other than in late gestation. Heifers may be infected in early gestation (Hillerton *et al.*, 1987). Spring calving heifers frequently become infected in the preceding autumn. Nationally, relatively few heifers are spring-calving so the incidence of infection is low and susceptibility may depend on whether an animal is pregnant or not and be less likely to change over pregnancy.

Age has a considerable effect on susceptibility to *A. pyogenes*/anaerobe mastitis (Hillerton, *et al.*, 1987). When the number of cases occurring in cows of particular ages is weighted according to the proportion of such animals in the herd it becomes apparent that cows in the fourth and subsequent lactations are more susceptible to *A. pyogenes*/anaerobe mastitis. The susceptibility apparently declines beyond lactation 6 and this may reflect relatively high disease resistance in those animals persisting longest in the herd. Considering the relatively high rate of infection established in heifers by experimental intramammary challenge these differences may reflect alterations in the resistance at the teat end brought about by milking.

Hillerton *et al.* (1987) have shown that infections occur most frequently in the front quarters of autumn calving cattle contrary to the situation with other forms of mastitis. The quarter distribution for *A. pyogenes*/anaerobe mastitis cases occurring at other times of the year is unknown. The former might reflect the easier access of flies to the teats and less disturbance from the tail.

It is most intriguing that when investigating field outbreaks of summer mastitis, neighbours, apparently farming in an identical manner, often never encounter summer mastitis problems. Local difference in pasture topography may be important (Hansen and Nielsen, 1983). Nutritional differences are less likely to be important as the problems are rarely on leys and major differences in disease incidence can occur *e.g.* in different groups of heifers on the same conserved downland. This circumstantial evidence supports either genetic variation in susceptibility, differences in attractiveness to a vector or micro-ecological differences between pastures. In all countries where the incidence of summer mastitis is high it is greater on low-lying, tree-lined meadows or leeward sides of hills than on more exposed pastures such as open downland. These local environments reflect the local climatic requirements of the supposed fly vector. Different types of pasture are more likely to affect the level of vector borne bacterial challenge to the cattle than by a manipulation of inherent susceptibility.

COINCIDENCES

A. pyogenes/anaerobe mastitis is a product of a series of events of varying probability. These include the extent and frequency of bacterial challenge, the susceptibility of the mammary gland to invasion and the subsequent likelihood of establishment of the bacteria. Environmental factors may influence these stages.

Challenge by the bacteria must be relatively common as all pathogens including the anaerobic bacteria are common around cattle and other species. Challenge may be increased as similar combinations of the bacteria occur in other infections. Investigation of the Veterinary Investigation Service returns in the U.K. shows that the seasonal peaks in *A. pyogenes* mastitis are coincident with peaks in foetopathy. In the U.K., cases of abortion are investigated closely but too few are diagnosed as being caused by *A. pyogenes* to produce a substantial increase in the environmental challenge by this organism.

In the summer the peak of *A. pyogenes*/anaerobe mastitis is coincident with the activity, specifically, of female *Hydrotaea irritans* on cattle and especially on their teats. Although this fly is widespread across the whole Palaearctic region it is not coincident with epidemic mastitis outside northern Europe. This may be attributed to the relatively low number of animals at risk in other areas, since all epidemic infections show some density dependence of host, *e.g.* in the Coruna region of Spain *H. irritans* occur on cattle but 70% of dairy cows calve in spring and less than 5% over the summer when the flies visit cattle (J. Rey, pers. comm.). This is probably similar for most other southern European countries. The fly is not found in Japan where an epidemic spread of the disease occurs in June. The commonest cattle-visiting fly there is *Musca hervei* but it has not been linked with the disease. Perhaps *H. meteorica*, shown to carry summer mastitis pathogens in the U.K. (Bramley *et al.*, 1985) and known to occur on cattle in Japan (H. Satashi, pers. comm.) is involved. In several developing world countries it is quite likely that an epidemic form of *A. pyogenes*/anaerobe mastitis occurs but is unrecognised because of its relatively low importance to the industry. Many of these countries have a high mastitis incidence and a large proportion of cows with a blind quarter.

It is difficult to find common features linking the two main disease episodes among housed cows in spring and pastured cattle in autumn other than late pregnancy. However at both these stages cattle are under environmental and nutritional stress.

Environmental stress affects the incidence of a variety of diseases in cattle and a long period of housing is a possible stressor similar to sustained fly pressure. In late winter cattle are under nutritional stress consuming possibly short supplies and late produced forage. Similarly in August pastures are often becoming bare, especially in the more marginal areas often used for dry cows and young stock.

It is worth considering, in conclusion, an epidemic outbreak of *A. pyogenes*/anaerobe mastitis which was reported from northern England in the winter/spring of 1986 (P.G. Francis, pers. comm.). Over 12 weeks, 112 quarters in lactating cows and a few in heifers became clinically infected. The infection involved *A. pyogenes, Peptostreptococcus indolicus* and microaerophilic cocci. There was some evidence of the involvement of *Mycoplasma californicum* too. The outbreak was progressive and the incidence, up to 58% attack rate, increased over the 12 weeks. This probably reflects a progressive fall in resistance of infection allied to a sustained or increasing bacterial challenge over the period. Initial faults in the milking machine related to excess vacuum, inadequate cleaning and pulsation were corrected and temporarily halted the occurrence of infection. The reduced resistance of cows has been ascribed to poor nutrition from high pH silage and low energy input. Infected and uninfected cattle moved to a different environment with improved hygiene, nutrition and husbandry suffered no further cases.

SUMMARY

A. pyogenes/anaerobe mastitis is most prevalent in pregnant, non-lactating, Friesian heifers and cows. The disease is endemic in northern Europe but particularly frequent in housed animals in spring and marked by severe outbreaks in July, August and September.

Summer outbreaks are coincident with the pestering of cattle by the fly *Hydrotaea irritans* which circumstantial evidence links with transmission of the disease. Various factors predispose to infection such as the age of cows, more exposed teats, teat and teat duct anatomy and possibly other genetic factors.

The influence of animal husbandry and the environment are poorly understood. Although disease can be controlled by rigorous pasture control and animal inspection it still occurs among cattle where rigorous fly control is practised or when flies cannot be implicated.

The effects of stress on the incidence of summer mastitis, in common with its effect on other infectious processes, is not understood. The effect of the environment as a whole, and nutrition on predisposition to infection, as well as genetic aspects, merit further consideration.

SUMMER MASTITIS IN IRISH DAIRY HERDS

W.J. Meaney* and J. Egan**

*An Foras Taluntais, Moorepark, Fermoy, Co. Cork, Ireland.
**The Veterinary Research Laboratory, Abbotstown, Castleknock, Dublin 15, Ireland.

ABSTRACT

Surveys in Irish dairy herds have shown that 6.7% of non-lactating cows and 3.0% of heifers developed clinical mastitis during the summer. Clinical mastitis was rarely encountered in non-lactating cows or heifers during the winter. Results from controlled experiments in spring calving animals, however, indicated that 10% of cows and 22.3% of heifers had clinical mastitis at calving.

Corynebacterium pyogenes and *Streptococcus dysgalactiae* were isolated from 31.7% and 39.9% of summer mastitis secretions respectively. In the same study, *Peptococcus indolicus* was present in 18.1% of secretions.

Results from spring calving animals showed that *C. pyogenes* and *Str. dysgalactiae* were cultured from 12.2% and 20.0% of secretions respectively.

INTRODUCTION

There are 1.58 million dairy cows in the Irish Republic and approximately 90% calve in springtime. Concern for clinical mastitis is, therefore mainly directed towards controlling environmental infection when animals are in winter housing. Problems relating to summer mastitis have generally been centred in two major liquid milk producing areas around Dublin and Cork. There are no statistics on the level of mastitis in the national dairy herd.

This report presents survey data on the incidence of summer mastitis in the major liquid milk producing areas. Data are also presented on the incidence of clinical mastitis in spring calving cows and heifers.

AUTUMN CALVING HERDS

Surveys carried out between 1978 and 1985 in a selected sample of 5,550 non-lactating cows and 3,426 heifers indicated that the mean incidence of clinical mastitis in cows and heifers was 6.7% and 3.0%, respectively (Table 1).

Infections occurred most frequently during the last week of July and the first 2 weeks of August each year. There were significantly ($p < 0.001$) more dry cows than heifers infected and the incidence in pregnant heifers was greater ($p < 0.001$) than in maiden heifers. The occurrence of infections in fore and hind udder quarters was similar.

TABLE 1. Prevalence of summer mastitis in selected herds

| Year | Number of susceptible animals | | Percentage of animals infected | |
	Cows	Heifers	Cows	Heifers
1978	440	N.R.*	10.0	
1979	1332	N.R.	5.0	
1980	1753	1135	5.1	2.4
1984	1207	1104	10.4	3.8
1985	818	1187	6.0	3.0
Total	5,550	3,426	6.7	3.0

*Not recorded.

Secretions from 193 clinical cases were cultured using aerobic and anaerobic bacteriological techniques. *Streptococcus dysgalactiae* and *Corynebacterium pyogenes* were the predominant bacteria isolated from the secretions (Table 2).

TABLE 2. Bacteria isolated from 193 summer mastitis secretions

| Bacterium | Number of secretions (%) | | |
	Pure culture	Mixed culture	Total
C. pyogenes	14 (7.3)	47 (24.4)	61 (31.7)
Str. dysgalactiae	24 (12.4)	53 (27.5)	77 (39.9)
Str. uberis	4 (2.1)	2 (1.0)	6 (3.1)
P. indolicus	2 (1.0)	33 (17.1)	35 (18.1)
S. aureus	6 (3.1)	21 (10.9)	27 (14.0)
Coliform	10 (5.2)	1 (0.5)	11 (5.7)
None isolated			28 (14.5)

SPRING CALVING HERDS

Clinical mastitis was studied in 8 herds over two non-lactating periods in 1362 cows and 547 heifers. At drying off, the cows were infused in all udder quarters with long acting antibiotic formulations. Animals were bedded on either clay, concrete, ground limestone or concrete covered with either ground limestone or hydrated lime. Foremilk quarter samples were collected aseptically from cows and heifers immediately after calving or at the first milking. Secretions were also collected from clinically affected quarters during the non-lactating period.

At calving, 10% of cows and 22.3% of heifers had clinical mastitis. Only 6 cases were detected prior to calving. Bacteriological results from the clinical secretions are summarised in Table 3. *Str. dysgalactiae*, aesculin positive streptococci and *C. pyogenes* were isolated from 20%, 11.3% and 12.2% of secretions respectively.

TABLE 3. **Bacteria isolated from 379 mastitis secretions in spring calving cows and heifers**

| | Number of clinical secretions | | | |
Bacterium	Cows	Heifers	Total	(%)
C. pyogenes	29	10	39	(10.3)
C. pyogenes/Str. dysgalactiae	1	1	2	(0.5)
C. pyogenes/Str. uberis	1	0	1	(0.3)
C. pyogenes/S. aureus	2	2	4	(1.1)
Str. dysgalactiae	21	53	74	(19.5)
Strep. (aesculin positive)	14	29	43	(11.3)
S. aureus	54	27	81	(21.4)
Coliform	29	24	53	(13.9)
Others	10	13	23	(6.1)
None isolated	23	36	59	(15.6)
Total	184	195	379	

RESULTS AND DISCUSSION

The survey results indicated that there were differences in the incidence of clinical mastitis in cows between years. The incidence was higher in cows than in heifers which was similar to reports from Great Britain (Marshall, 1981). Higher levels were recorded in heifers in other studies (O'Rourke *et al.*, 1985; Franke *et al.*, 1983).

Streptococcus dysgalactiae and *Corynebacterium pyogenes* were the most frequently isolated bacteria and were predominantly in mixed culture. In this survey, the samples were collected by the herdsmen and this may have contributed to the high frequency of mixed culture. However, in a study by Sol *et al.* (1985) where samples were collected by veterinarians a similar pattern emerged.

In spring calving animals, 10% of cows and 22.3% of heifers were clinically affected at calving. Most of the bacterial isolates were in pure culture. Sampling was carried out by trained technicians but secretions were not cultured anaerobically. Forty-four percent of infections were associated with either *C. pyogenes, Str. dysgalactiae* or other aesculin positive streptococci.

The level of *C. pyogenes* infections in spring was approximately one third of the level recorded in autumn but was similar to the level of gram negative infections in spring.

Treatment with antibiotics had little effect in controlling *C. pyogenes* infections or preventing losses of udder quarters. *C. pyogenes* has been isolated from various sites in cattle, including the reproductive tract (Lovell 1943; Sorensen, 1976; Hartigan, 1980). Infected discharges, therefore, increase the bacterial challenge, especially in animals confined during the winter and may be a factor associated with the incidence of *C. pyogenes* infection in spring.

A close association has been established between *C. pyogenes* and *Str. dysgalactiae* in the pathogenesis of summer mastitis (Schwan and Holmberg, 1978/79). In Ireland, streptococci (*dysgalactiae* and aesculin positive strains) have been the most frequently isolated bacterial types from clinical secretions in autumn and spring calving animals.

The aetiology of *C. pyogenes*, *Str. dysgalactiae* and other aesculin positive streptococci requires further investigation particularly in relation to spring calving animals.

THE OCCURRENCE OF SUMMER MASTITIS RELATED TO THE FORAGING ACTIVITIES OF *HYDROTAEA IRRITANS* (FALL.)

Soren Achim Nielsen*, B. Overgaard Nielsen**, J.W. Hansen***,
P. Nansen*** and J. Olesen****

*Institute of Biology and Chemistry, Roskilde University, Roskilde, Denmark.
**The Zoological Laboratory, University of Aarhus, Aarhus, Denmark.
***Institute of Hygiene and Microbiology, Royal Veterinary and Agricultural University, Copenhagen, Denmark.
****Agrometeorological Service, Danish Research Service for Plant and Soil Science, Research Centre Foulum, Denmark.

ABSTRACT

The incidence of summer mastitis was studied as a function of climatic fluctuations and fluctuations in the foraging activity of *Hydrotaea irritans* in order to evaluate the possible role of the fly as a vector of the disease. The results obtained supported the assumption that *Hydrotaea irritans* was a causative link in the transmission of summer mastitis.

INTRODUCTION

Olesen *et al.* (1985) demonstrated that variation in the incidence of summer mastitis corresponded to climatic oscillations. Nielsen *et al.* (1983) showed that the foraging activities of the plantation fly *Hydrotaea irritans* was related to climatic conditions and the incidence of summer mastitis. In this paper we shall look at the spatio-temporal relations between the rate of fly attack and climatic conditions in an attempt to prove an expected causal connection between fly attack and summer mastitis incidence.

MATERIAL AND METHODS

The investigation was carried out in 1981 at Store Vildmose in the northern part of Jutland, Denmark. About 3000 heifers graze in this area every year and these are examined daily for different diseases, including summer mastitis.

Hydrotaea irritans was collected from heifers twice a day at 10 a.m. and at 3 p.m. during the season when the fly was active. The collection was carried out by means of a vacuum cleaner at two different locations, the head and udder, for 3 minutes in each locality. Synchronously, the following variables were measured: air temperature, relative humidity, wind direction and force, cloudiness and precipitation. The quantitative relations between plantation fly attacks and climatic fluctuations were examined by means of simple correlation and multiple regression analyses (Draper and Smith, 1966) and analysis of varience (ANOVA) after log transformation of fly numbers.

RESULTS

Table 1 shows the squares of the correlation coefficient for different climatic variables on fly attack ratio. The variables measured, except for cloudiness, affected the estimation of fly attack significantly ($p < 0.001$) and all variables are more or less intercorrelated. The parameter estimates were positive for air temperature and humidity and negative for wind velocity. Fluctuations in air temperature and wind velocity are the most important. The total effect of the four variables (Table 1) included in the test explains 19.5% of the attacks on the head and 23.7% on the udder region ($p < 0.0001$).

When precipitation conditions were included in the calculations (see Table 2) 26.2 and 31.3% of the fly attacks were explained for the head and udder regions, respectively (ANOVA: $p < 0.001$).

TABLE 1. The relation between the number of foraging *H. irritans* on the 2 body regions and climatic parameters: the effect of adding the different variables on cumulative r^2 (square of the correlation coefficient).

	Air Temp. r^2	Wind force r^2	Rel. hum. r^2	Cloudiness r^2	Total r^2	Significance
Head region	0.119	0.188	0.194	0.195	0.195	< 0.001
Udder region	0.186	0.233	0.235	0.237	0.237	< 0.001

TABLE 2. The relation between the number of foraging *H. irritans* on the 2 body regions and climatic parameters: the effect of including precipitation on cumulative r^2.

	Total r^2 for air temp. + wind force + rel. hum. + cloudiness	r^2 for air temp. + rel. hum. + wind force + cloudiness + precipitation	r^2 for air temp. + wind force + precipitation
Head region	0.195	0.296	0.262
Udder region	0.237	0.339	0.313

In Table 3 the effects of temperature and wind velocity calculated from the regression coefficients are expressed as the values necessary to double and halve the fly attack. These values are given separately for head and udder regions.

Attack activity is halved in both head and udder regions by a rise in wind velocity of about 3.5 m.s^{-1}. There is a difference between the head and udder regions in the amount of increase necessary to result in doubling on fly attack in both air temperature and relative humidity. A rise of only about 3.5°C in air temperature will double attacks in the udder region but it requires approximately 5.5°C to obtain the same effect in the head region. Similarly, whereas an increase of 49.5% in humidity of sufficient to double fly attack in the head region, a rise of 63.01% is required in the udder region.

TABLE 3.   The effect of changes in climatic conditions on activity of *H. irritans* expressed as the amount of increase in specific climatic variables necessary to double or halve the attack rate on head and udder regions.

| | Doubling of activity | | Halving of activity |
	Air temp. in °C	Rel. humidity in %	Wind force in m.s^{-1}
Head region	5.29	49.51	3.75
Udder region	3.32	63.01	3.43

DISCUSSION

Day to day fluctuations in climatic variables are of importance in the activity pattern of *H. irritans*. Air temperature, wind force and precipitation are especially important factors. However, other climatic conditions, which are more or less intercorrelated with the above mentioned variables, are also of significance.

Air temperature, wind force and precipitation explain about 26% and 31% of fly attacks in the head and udder regions, respectively (Table 2). This indicates that the activity observed includes both non-biotic and biotic aspects. Table 3 shows that a relatively small increase in wind force reduces foraging activity. Moreover, wind force influences the rate of fly attack equally in both head and udder regions. One explanation for this could be that the general flight activity of the flies is lowered by the influence of wind.

Variations in air temperature could explain the difference in the number of *H. irritans* foraging on the head and udder region. The rationale underlying this is as follows. *H. irritans* is unable to penetrate undamaged skin of cattle independently. However, a proportionally heavier attack by *H. irritans* could be provoked by a relatively heavier attack of tiny biting flies (Ceratopogonidae: *Culicoides* spp.) and blackflies (Simuliidae) which attack grazing cattle in large numbers. The members of the latter two dipteran groups are more sensitive to low air temperatures and risies in wind velocity than *H. irritans*. Nielsen (1982) calculated the average value for doubling the flight activity of the different species of bitting midges attacking pastured cattle to be 2.85°C. Moreover, most of these actively blood-sucking species prefer foraging on the belly and udder regions of cattle. This could thus explain the proportional increase of *H. irritans* foraging on the udder region with rising temperature as this non-biting species is attracted by wounds made by the actively biting diptera.

In 1986 the distribution of summer mastitis incidences in Store Vildmose deviated greatly from normal as the largest incidence was recorded early in summer (mid-July).

This deviation could be explained by the prior 10 day period of heavy *H. irritans* attack. The results of Olesen *et al.* (1985) indicate a relation between the appearance of summer mastitis and periods with high air temperature and low wind velocity. Their finding of a time lag of 10 days between periods with favourable climatic conditions and waves of summer mastitis is in agreement with the present findings regarding the activity pattern of *H. irritans* in varying climatic conditions. The results of these investigations confirm the assumption that *Hydrotaea irritans* is an important vector of summer mastitis.

ACKNOWLEDGEMENTS

We are greatly indebted to Professor Jorgen Clausen and Secretary Inger Johansen, Univ. of Roskilde, Denmark for reading and criticising the manuscript. The study was financially supported by the Danish Agricultural and Veterinary Research Council.

HEIFER MASTITIS IN SWEDEN DURING A THREE YEAR PERIOD (1982 – 1985): BACKGROUND AND SOME PRELIMINARY DATA ON THE INCIDENCE OF HEIFER MASTITIS

S-O. Olsson*, P. Jonsson**/***, O. Holmberg**/**** and H. Funke*

*Swedish Association for Livestock Breeding and Production, Animal Health Department, S-631 84 Eskilstuna, Sweden.
**National Veterinary Institute, Uppsala, Sweden.
***Present address: Ewos AB, Box 618, S-151 27 Södertälje, Sweden.
****Swedish University of Agricultural Sciences, Department of Veterinary Microbiology, Section of Clinical Microbiology, Uppsala, Sweden.

ABSTRACT

Heifer mastitis has been known in Sweden for a long time. Records of the disease go back as far as the 1920's. In 1953 a report was published on the prevalence of mastitis among heifers and dry cows during one summer in a county in southern Sweden. In 1972 – 1976 an investigation was carried out on the island of Gotland, in which it was found that annually 8 – 10% of the heifers on the island were affected. Based on various trials and reports from farmers and veterinarians, a nation-wide survey was made in 1982 – 1985 on the incidence of heifer mastitis, infection pattern, influence of environment and management factors, the importance of the insect fauna, as well as certain trials involving prophylactic measures. A preliminary report on the frequency of heifer mastitis in five out of eight trial areas is presented together with the monthly distribution of the cases. The number of cases per herd is also shown. The results are discussed and put in relation to earlier Swedish investigations.

INTRODUCTION

This report briefly describes earlier Swedish investigations of heifer mastitis. A study covering a period of three years is presented together with some preliminary data on the occurrence of heifer mastitis in Sweden.

Heifer mastitis was described in Sweden more than thirty years ago (Niléhn and Niléhn, 1953). Records on the disease can be found as far back as the 1920's. The authors describe mastitis in grazing, pregnant and non-pregnant heifers and dry cows under the designation pasture or summer mastitis. By means of an inquiry to the veterinary practitioners in the country of Malmöhus a total of 971 cases was reported, 549 of which were in heifers. One hundred and sixty of the heifers were not mated.

In 1972 – 1976 a study on heifer mastitis was carried out on the island of Gotland (Everz and Linge, 1979). Annually 15 – 20% of the herds exhibited one or several cases of heifer mastitis. Each year 8 – 10% of the heifers on the island caught the disease. Fifty to sixty percent of the diseased animals were slaughtered, approximately 30% yielded only on three quarters, while 10 – 20% recovered after veterinary treatment. No concentration of heifer mastitis to a certain type of biotope could be established in the trial. Most cases were discovered in August and September.

In 1980 an inquiry was made in south-east Sweden (the area of Kalmar) and Gotland regarding the incidence of heifer mastitis during 1979. Five percent of the heifers on Gotland and 3% in the Kalmar area had heifer mastitis. Fifty-eight percent of the cases occurred in the period July to October. Fifty percent of the cases were discovered in the last month of pregnancy (Pettersson, 1980).

Based on the above mentioned investigations from the 1970's and a continuously growing number of reports both from veterinarians and farmers on increasing problems with heifer mastitis, a comprehensive study on heifer mastitis in Sweden was initiated in 1982 by the Swedish Association for Livestock Breeding and Production and the National Veterinary Institute. The project is described below together with some preliminary data on the incidence of heifer mastitis in different parts of Sweden.

The following definition of heifer mastitis was agreed on at a Nordic heifer mastitis seminar and was used in this investigation: "The comprehensive term for all inflammatory reactions developed in the udder of female cattle in the period from the onset of puberty to a fortnight after the first calving. Simultaneously, we must recognize that it is only possible to diagnose cases of heifer mastitis with clinical symptoms". (Klastrup, 1979).

PROJECT PLAN

The aim of the investigation, which was carried out from July 1st 1982 until the 31st October 1985 was study the frequency of heifer mastitis, the infection pattern and the variation in different parts of Sweden as well as the relation to different environment and management factors. The effect of certain prophylactic measures was also studied.

Eight veterinary districts were selected to represent various geographic regions in Sweden and also with regard to the type of biotope and the occurrence of heifer mastitis.

The investigation comprised the following parts:

- Bacteriological examination of clinical cases.
- Survey of the frequency of heifer mastitis in milk-recorded herds.
- Detailed studies in certain herds with regard to environment and management.
- Study of the insect fauna on the pastures under different environmental conditions.
- Bacteriological examination of foremilk samples from heifers within 1 — 7 days calving in order to study the occurrence of subclinical heifer mastitis.
- Trials with certain prophylactic measures (teat sealing, insect repellants).

MATERIAL

Data on reported cases of heifer mastitis were collected each month from all milk-recorded herds in the eight trial areas. Notes were made on the identity of each diseased animal. The recordings, which are normally not included in the routines of the milk-recording staff, were made on regular milk-recording visits.

RESULTS AND DISCUSSION

Preliminary results from five trial areas are shown in Table 1.

TABLE 1. Number of cases of heifer mastitis reported from milk-recorded herds from 01-07-1982 to 31-12-1985 and the average frequency of affected herds and heifers during the same period of time.

| | | | | | Frequency (%) | |
| | | | | | Affected | Heifer |
Area	1982	1983	1984	1985	herds	mastitis
Hörby	79	69	42	30	22	2.4
Falkenberg	57	113	170	147	32	4.6
Arvika/Årjäng	9	50	43	45	18	2.9
Jämtland	9	47	33	13	9	1.1
Ångermanland	14	26	19	7	9	1.5
Total	168	305	307	242	19	2.7

Table 2 shows the percentage distribution of reported cases per calendar month.

TABLE 2. Percentage distribution of reported cases of heifer mastitis from 01-07-1982 to 31-12-1985 per calendar month.

January	5%	July	2%
February	4%	August	18%
March	4%	September	22%
April	3%	October	16%
May	1%	November	13%
June	1%	December	11%

Table 3 shows the number of reported cases per herd in three trial areas from 01-07-1982 to 31-12-1985.

TABLE 3.   Number of reported cases per herd in three trial areas from
                              01-07-1982 to 31-12-1985.

Number of reported cases per herd	Number of cases per group	% of the total number of reported cases
1	380	68
2	103	19
3	46	8
4	12	2
≥ 5	14	3

The frequency of heifer mastitis in this preliminary report is equivalent to that found in two other Swedish investigations. A study in south-east Sweden reported an average of 4% (Pettersson, 1980). The frequency of heifer mastitis in an area in south-west Sweden was 2.7% (Wass, 1986). In an earlier investigation on Gotland a frequency of 8 − 10% was reported (Everz and Linge, 1979). Even though all collected data have not yet been processed, the frequency of heifer mastitis seems to be relatively low in Sweden. However, the number of affected herds is comparatively high and seems to be higher in southern than in northern Sweden. The earlier mentioned reports from farmers and veterinarians on increasing problems with heifer mastitis may be caused by an increase in the number of affected herds.

Fifty-six percent of the cases were reported during the period August − October. However, milk-recorded herds are not visited by the field recorders during July and thus most July cases were recorded in August. Sixty-one percent of the cases were discovered during the first week after calving (day of calving included) according to an examination of cases which have been bacteriologically analysed (Jonsson et al, 1986). As autumn calving is common in Sweden this may partly explain the seasonal clustering of cases. Forty-four percent of the heifers calve during the same period of time. For additional studies of the seasonal variation, the material will be further processed with a view to the distribution of calving over the year.

Heifer mastitis seems to occur mostly as isolated cases in a herd. Coinciding cases in the same herd are more rare. The data shows that 68% of reported cases are single cases in a herd. Only 5% of the cases relate to herds which have reported more than four cases per year. It should however be pointed out that the average number of cows in Swedish milk-recorded herds is approximately 25, which means that the average herd has 8 − 10 pregnant heifers. One or two cases of heifer mastitis can therefore be regarded as quite a serious problem for a individual farmer. Even though the frequency of heifer mastitis as a whole is fairly low, the economic importance of the disease should be further evaluated.

ACKNOWLEDGEMENTS

The Farmers' Research Council for Information and Development financially supported this work.

THE EPIDEMIOLOGY OF SUMMER MASTITIS IN THE NETHERLANDS

J. Sol*, U. Vecht** and J.W. Seinhorst***

*Animal Health Service Institute in Overijssel and Flevoland,
Postbus 13, 8000 AA Zwolle, The Netherlands.
**Dept. of Bacteriology, Central Veterinary Institute, Lelystad, The Netherlands.
***Proefstation v.d. Rundveehouderij, Lelystad, The Netherlands.

ABSTRACT

Summer mastitis is an acute mastitis which is only seen in the summer months in pastured, non-lactating cattle, *i.e.*, dry cows, heifers and calves. The clinical signs and isolated bacteria are typical and must be seperated from other mastitis cases in dry cattle in summer or winter time. The disease is enzootic in certain areas in the Netherlands but only sporadic in others. Soil and vegetation (trees and bushes) are important but summer mastitis is also seen in quite open areas without trees and bushes. The role of *H. irritans* in the etiology seems to be important. The incidence of summer mastitis varies between years and has, for the last 3 years, been as low as 0.2%. This is probably the reason that over 50% of the acute mastitis cases in dry cattle could not be confirmed bacteriologically as summer mastitis in 1984 and 1985. In 1980 the incidence on the same farms was as high as 10%. Calves contract less summer mastitis than heifers. The highest incidence rate is seen in dry cows which also have the most serious clinical symptoms. Pregnancy seems to have no influence. Cows still with a high milk yield at drying off are more susceptible to summer mastitis. If there is a calf, heifer or cow which sucks other cattle the incidence of summer mastitis rises dramatically in a herd. There is no difference in susceptibility between the various breeds in the Netherlands but the Jersey which is said to be rather insusceptible is hardly seen in Holland. There are, however, heritable differences. Daughters of bulls with a high peak milk flow are more susceptible, as are daughters of easy milking cows. This is probably the reason why heifers from certain farms contract more summer mastitis than heifers from other farms at the same time in the same pasture. Front quarters are twice as much affected as hind quarters with summer mastitis. Front and hind quarters are equally affected in acute mastitis in dry cattle during the summer which is caused by other bacteria than those typical for summer mastitis.

DEFINITION OF SUMMER MASTITIS

A well described definition of summer mastitis is essential for a responsible epidemiology. In the Netherlands summer mastitis is considered to be an enzootic, acute udder infection that occurs in non-lactating, pastured cattle during the summer. The infected quarter is painfull, swollen and hard. The secretion is usually thick, yellowish green, sometimes contains blood and has an unpleasant, typical odour. The infected animal usually has a fever, is anorexic, a raised abdomen and walks stiffly because of the septicaemia (Saes, 1971).

The infected quarter is usually lost to milk production. The animal often suffers severe loss of weight or is slaughtered.

The bacteria which are considered to be typical for summer mastitis are: *Corynebacterium pyogenes, Peptococcus indolicus* and a microaerophilic coc also referred to as the Stuart-Schwan coc. *P. indolicus* is considered to be responsible for the the typical odour (Sol, 1985). A large number of other bacteria have also been isolated from infections. These include *Fusobacterium necrophorum, Bacteroides melaninogenicus, Bacillus* spp., *Streptococcus uberis, Streptococcus dysgalactiae* (particularly in dry cows in the U.K.), Staphylococcae, etc. (Tolle *et al.*, 1985).

In many countries summer mastitis is also used to describe the udder infection found in heifers in or near the first week of calving for the first time. This is also observed in the Netherlands. The clinical symptoms of these infections deviates considerably from those of summer mastitis. Although the udder is always swollen it is softer. The secretion is usually whitish-yellow, thin and lumpy and lacks the typical odour. Treatment is usually successful. These infections are seen in the summer but more in the winter. Although usually involving one animal on a farm sometimes many are affected within a short time. The bacteria isolated are often coliform, staphylococcae and streptococcae. Typical summer mastitis bacteria are rarely isolated. Similar infections are also seen in 1—2 year old heifers both in summer and winter. The infections are often confused with summer mastitis by farmers.

Udder infections in dry cows also make up a special group. They are frequently caused by *S. uberis, S. agalactiae,* staphyloccoae *etc.* and are seen both in winter and summer. Summer mastitis is also found in dry cows but is difficult to distinguish from *e.g.* a *S. dysgalactiae* infection on clinical grounds (Weitz, 1949). Francis *et al.* (1986) reported a peak in *C. pyogenes* mastitis in March particularly in dry cows in autumn calving herds. The total mastitis incidence was also high in this study in January, February and March but no statistical tests were applied to determine if the March peak differed significantly from other months.

C. pyogenes mastitis is also seen in the Netherlands particularly in the winter, both in dry and lactating cows. This "Winter *C. pyogenes* mastitis" can be generally traced back to teat injuries. *C. pyogenes* mastitis is rarely seen in lactating cows which do not have teat damage. Clinical mastitis caused by *C. pyogenes* in lactating cows in the winter is also reported from Ireland but this *C. pyogenes* mastitis is usually proceeded by a mastitis caused by other bacteria, usually streptococcae (Egan, 1985). In Holland, the use of the term summer mastitis with respect to cows is confined to that group which is pastured, dry and have no teat damage. Even here there is a large chance of confusion with *S. dysgalactiae* mastitis unless bacteriological tests are made to confirm the diagnosis.

In view of the above ambiguousness regarding udder infections and given the frequent presence of *C. pyogenes* and/or anaerobes, it was decided at the Heifer Mastitis Symposium held at Stockholm/Helsinki in 1983 to refer to the infection as summer mastitis if this involved a *C. pyogenes*/anaerobic syndrome in animals up to the first calving in the summer and distinguish it from *C. pyogenes* mastitis in cows and heifers that had calved (Saes, 1983).

DISTRIBUTION OF SUMMER MASTITIS

Summer mastitis occurs enzootically in Sweden, Denmark, West and East Germany, the Netherlands, Belgium, England, Ireland and Scotland. Incidental cases are also reported from other countries.

In the Netherlands large differences are present between different areas (Saes, 1971; Sol, 1983). It is not seen in some areas whereas in others it is common. Summer mastitis occurs primarily on sandy soils (7.2%) less on marshy soil (5.3%) and hardly ever on clay (1.2%) (Sol, 1983). The typical biotope appears to be sandy or lowlying, wooded land with poor drainage. In Holland, as in Denmark, summer mastitis can also occur in open, non-wooded areas and direct access to water is not essential.

Summer mastitis may occur year after year on some farms but is, in any particular year, unpredictable. Similarly, comparison with neighbouring pastures is also impossible (Sol and Vardy, 1982; Sol, 1983).

TIME OF OCCURRENCE

The summer mastitis season in the Netherlands begins in June and ends in September except for incidental cases in October. Approximately 4% of cases occur in June, 90% in July and August (with a peak between 15 July and 15 August) and the remaining 6% in September and October (Sol, 1983).

Summer mastitis occurs mostly in warm, humid weather usually shortly after a temperature increase to 30°C (Sol, 1983).

The peak incidence can also vary within the season. When a summer mastitis case occurs, one or more new cases are seen a few days later in 35% of the herds, independent of herd size (Sol, 1983).

INCIDENCE OF SUMMER MASTITIS

The incidence of summer mastitis in the Netherlands varies considerably between years as may be seen in Table 1.

An explanation for the low summer mastitis incidence in the Netherlands over recent years (Table 1) is difficult as this is also true for farms where no preventive measures have been taken. It can be said that fly control methods are more efficient *e.g.* in 1985 and 1986, 66% of the farms in summer mastitis areas made use of ear tags. Moreover, in 1983 and 1984 the springs tended to be cold and wet. A low incidence of summer mastitis in these years has also been recorded in Denmark (Annual Report of the Danish Pest Infestation Laboratory, 1984 and 1985) and Schleswig Holstein (Tolle *et al.*, 1985). This was less evident in England (O'Rourke *et al.*, 1984).

Approximately 70% of the 500,000 heifers in the Netherlands are pastures in "summer mastitis areas". This means that the incidence in heifers in recent years has varied between

± 35,000 cases in 1980 to ± 1,000 in 1985.

TABLE 1. Incidence of summer mastitis in 1—2 year old heifers in Overijssel, the Netherlands. The data are taken from 198 farms.

	Year							
	1979	1980	1981	1982	1983	1984	1985	1986
Number of heifers	3290	3706	3959	3832	3989	3957	3912	
% summer mastitis	9.5	10.0	3.4	4.1	1.1	0.2	0.2	~ 0.2

TRANSMISSION OF SUMMER MASTITIS

It is generally accepted that summer mastitis is transmitted by the fly *Hydrotaea irritans*. Only in England have successful transmission experiments using *H. irritans* been described (Tarry, 1978).

H. irritans is sometimes frequently seen on particular meadows wheras it is almost or completely absent on adjoining, otherwise identical ones. *H. irritans* is the fly seen most frequently on the udder and, because it is fairly mobile and forages everywhere, is the fly most contaminated with bacteria (Bramley *et al.*, 1985; Sorensen, 1974). *Haematobia irritans* which is often seen on the teat in lying animals is far less contaminated. A subclinical *C. pyogenes* mastitis may be found in 9% of heifers (Bock, 1980). It is possible that additional bacteria may give rise to the typical summer mastitis syndrome.

DIFFERENCES BETWEEN ANIMALS

Lactation phase. Summer mastitis is only found in non-lactating animals.

Age. The influence of age on the chance of having summer mastitis is a controversial issue. Saes (1971) found no difference in the incidence in calves and heifers pastured on the same meadows in the Netherlands. Tolle *et al.* (1985) on the other hand found large differences between calves, heifers and cows. Similar differences have also been found in the Netherlands (Table 2).

It should be stated, however, that since the early seventies, most calves are not pastured before July and that many are never turned out. In addition to this, calves have small teats which are often thickly imbedded in hair. Summer mastitis is also rarely seen in calves in England (Bramley *et al.*, 1977).

Summer mastitis is often seen in cows during the summer. According to Weitz (1949), the incidence in "at risk" individuals in England can reach 25%. Moreover, Weitz states that older cows are more at risk, but these also have sub-clinical mastitis more frequently. Weitz also found more summer mastitis just after drying off and shortly before calving. It is possible that a sub-clinical mastitis predisposes the development of a typical summer mastitis if flies have free access to the udder. This is the case if no insecticides are used.

TABLE 2.   **Summer mastitis incidence in 1980 on 844 farms in Overijssel (data from Sol, 1983).**

Category	Number	% summer mastitis
Dry and lactating cows	42,894	1.46
Heifers	14,480	5.83
Calves	15,998	0.74

The incidence in dry cows in the Netherlands, if consideration is taken of the fact that they are only 6—8 weeks "at risk" during the dry period, in 1980 was ± 10% (Sol, 1983).

If correction is made for the number of dry cows "at risk" then the summer mastitis percentage in this category is approximately twice that of heifers. The same is true for Germany (Tolle et al., 1985) if this was corrected using the same criteria as in the Netherlands.

TABLE 3.   **Percentage summer mastitis in dry cows in 1980 on 844 farms in Overijssel and comparable data form England (taken from O'Rourke et al., 1984) and Germany (taken from Tolle et al., 1985).**

Category	Netherlands	England	West Germany
Cows	1.46	0.5	2.0
Corrected for dry cows only	±9.0	1.5	±11.0
Heifers	5.83	1.3	5.8
Calves	0.74	—	1.1

Pregnancy. If is often reported that pregnant animals are more prone to summer mastitis. However, in the majority of publications it is generally ignored that in summer most heifers are a few months pregnant in July and August. Knoef (1981) found a difference in relative incidence between 1—1½ and 1½—2 year old heifers of 12.3% and 18%, respectively. In the > 2 year group the relative incidence was 16.5%. Knoef's material was selected, as cases were reported by veterinarians. A farmer will call the vet more quickly when the animal has been pregnant for some time than for a non-pregnant heifer. Schmolt et al. (1974) found no difference between 12—15 and 18—20 month old heifers. Saes (1971) found no infuence of pregnancy on incidence. Reports from Denmark (Annual Report DPIL, 1984, 1985) indicate a higher incidence in pregnant animals but a further analysis has yet to come.

Dry cows. Cows that are dried off while still giving much milk are more sensitive to summer mastitis. Such cows are, in general, predisposed to catch mastitis. This problem exists currently in the Netherlands as cows are dried off earlier because of the supertax on milk production. This led to serious outbreaks on two farms in 1986, in one case 40 of the 72 dry cows became infected with summer mastitis.

Suckers. The presence of suckers in a herd causes a problem in that more summer mastitis occurs. Pearson (1951) reported two summer mastitis cases with a farmer who continued stripping his cows after drying off.

Breed differences. Differences in susceptibility exist between different breeds. The Angler, Jersey and Red Danish breeds are less susceptable than FH/HF cows (Tolle *et al.*, 1985). This makes it more remarkable that Tarry (1978) obtained summer mastitis in 2 out of 8 Jersey cows in transmission experiments with *H. irritans*.

Influence of the mother. Daughters of mothers which are light milkers are more susceptible than those from medium to difficult to milk cows as can be seen in Tables 4 and 5.

TABLE 4.   Relation between ease of milking in the mother and summer mastitis in the daughter (after Knoef, 1981).

Ease of milking	Number of animals	N. summer mastitis cases	%
Difficult	41	2	4.9
Normal	950	147	15.5
Easy	101	32	31.7
Unknown	923	137	14.8

TABLE 5.   Relation between ease of milking of the mother and summer mastitis in the daughter (data taken from Dommerholt, 1985).

Ease of milking in mother;	N	(%)	Summer mastitis (16 animals)	
Difficult	444	(9.4)	0	(0%)
Normal	3510	(74.5)	12	(75%)
Easy	763	(16.2)	4	(25%)

Influence of the bull. Offspring of bulls with a high milking speed are more susceptible to summer mastitis (Knoef, 1981).

Influence of the farm. In meadows where heifers from different farms are pastured together it is often found that summer mastitis cases are clustered in animals from particular farms. This may be partly due to genetic factors.

Fore and hind quarters. Opinions regarding differences in susceptibility between fore and quarters are contradictory in the literature. Sorensen (1974) found no differences. Knoef (1981) examined data on 322 cases treated by veterinarians on 241 farms. The data are given in Table 6 and show that summer mastitis occurs twice as frequently in fore quarters.

TABLE 6.   Incidence of summer mastitis in different quarters.

	Right fore	Left fore	Right hind	Left hind	2 quarters	3 quarters
N. animals	101	100	50	46	23	2
% summer mastitis	31	31	16	14	7	1

Number of teats affected. Knoef also found that in 8% of the cases 2 or more quarters were infected. Saes (1971) arrived at a slightly higher percentage, 11.1% in 306 animals.

Hairiness of the teat. Over, quoted in Sol (1983), reported that teats that are covered with thick hair are less likely to be affected by summer mastitis. Similarly, Groothuis states that such teats are less prone to fly bites (Sol, 1983).

PROGNOSIS OF SUMMER MASTITIS

Cows are generally more sick than heifers and the latter more sick than calves. Cows occassionally die whereas this is rarely seen in heifers and calves.

DIAGNOSIS OF SUMMER MASTITIS

In recent years in the Netherlands it appears that more than 50% of the acute udder infections in dry cattle during the summer reported by farmers cannot, bacteriologically be classified as summer mastitis (Sol *et al.*, 1985). These udder infections may be classified as Category III (Sol *et al.*, 1985). Acute mastitis cases in dry cattle during the summer which are treated by veterinarians on request of the farmer are in 80% of the cases, bacteriologically classified as summer mastitis.

METHOD OF PREVENTION

Even if ear-tags are utilized udder infections may still occur. However, these usually involve infections from which non-typical summer mastitis bacteria are isolated and where fore and hind quarters are equally frequently affected (Dommerholt, 1985).

ACKNOWLEDGEMENTS

We would like to thank the National Animal Health Committee, The Hague and the Central Veterinary Institute for their support of the summer mastitis project.

FACTORS CONTRIBUTING TO DIFFERENTIAL RISK BETWEEN HEIFERS IN CONTRACTING SUMMER MASTITIS

G. Thomas*,**, H.J. Prijs* and J.J. Trapman**

*Dept. of Parasitology, Central Veterinary Institute,
Postbox 65, 8200 AB Lelystad, The Netherlands.
**Dept. of Animal Physiology, University of Groningen,
Postbox 14, 9750 AA Haren, The Netherlands.

ABSTRACT

A survey is given of factors which may contribute to differential risk between heifers in contracting summer mastitis. These include such aspects as genetic background and the physiological condition of the individual. As yet very little attention has been paid to the causal factors which lead to increased risk. One aspect that has been largely ignored is the cause underlying relative differences in attractiveness to flies, particularly *Hydrotaea irritans* and the accompanying increase in probability of transmission. Data are given which indicate that odour signals emanating from the individual contribute to differential risk.

INTRODUCTION

It is commonly reported in the literature that the risk in contracting summer mastitis is not equal for all individuals. Some of the host factors that have been suggested as underlying this differential in risk are summarised in Table 1.

TABLE 1.   **Host factors which have been associated with differential risk.**

Genetic backgroud

Breed

Sire, dam (light milking)

Morphological, physiological and behavioural aspects

Physiological condition — age, reproductive status, general condition.

Fly access — differences in morphology of teat and opening, hairiness, effectiveness of fly
        dislodging behaviour.

As far as genetic background is concerned, several publications have indicated differences in summer mastitis incidence between breeds. Schwan (1979) states that the majority of cases in Sweden occur in the Swedish Friesian breed despite the predominance of the Swedish Red and White. In Denmark, the RDM breed appears to be more at risk than the SDM or Jersey breeds (Sorensen, 1974; Hansen and Nielsen, 1983). Both Black and Red

Friesians have a higher incidence than Angler cattle in Schleswig-Holstein (Franke *et al.*, 1983). Genetic crossing of high and low susceptible breeds has, in one instance at least, led to a reduction in incidence (Muller, 1977). Genetically linked differences in susceptibility have also been suggested to operate at the individual level within breeds. Two factors that have been particularly implicated are influence of sire (Hansen and Nielsen, 1983) and whether or not the dam is an easy milker (Knoef, quoted in Sol, 1983).

Differences in risk have also been correlated with a specific physiological condition of the individual. Some of the important variables here are age (Wennemar, 1974; Sorensen, 1974; Bjorn *et al.*, 1985), pregnancy status (Hansen and Nielsen, 1983) and lactation phase (Heidrich *et al.*, 1964).

Although the above factors can be correlated to differential risk in contracting summer mastitis they do not, in themselves, help to explain the causes of these differences in individual risk. For this, the answers must be sought in three areas:

1. the resistance of the individual to infection
2. differences between hosts in ease of access to potential infection sites for fly vectors and the pathogenes they carry, and
3. relative differences between hosts in their attraction for vectors, leading to higher fly pestation and thus increased probability of transmission.

The first of these is beyond the scope of this paper and will not be considered further. Both (2) and (3) involve host/vector interactions which is one of the concentration areas in the extant dutch summer mastitis project.

Some of the factors which are important in determining differences between hosts in ease of access to potential infection sites have been indicated in Table 1. These include differences in morphology of the teat duct and its opening (Hansen and Nielsen, 1983) and the presence or absence of the teat duct plug (Nielsen). The hairiness of the teat and udder also plays a role in that reduced hair density and/or length allows easier access to the foraging fly (Nielsen, 1985; Prijs, pers. obs.). Another factor which is probably of importance here is the efficiency of the fly dislodging behaviour of the individual heifer.

As yet, almost no research has been carried out on relative differences between hosts in their attraction for vectors and the consequent effect on differential risk. We have recently started a research programme into these differences particularly with respect to their causality.

MATERIAL AND METHODS

The research was carried out using 4 test herds (K, E, W and A) in the province of Overijssel, the Netherlands. These were followed over the whole summer season and flies were counted several times weekly on all animals.

RESULTS AND DISCUSSION

It has long been known that fly load varies between individual cattle. Moreover, these individual differences tend to remain constant not only over the whole season but can also persist between seasons. Figure 1 gives an example of this phenomenon. One individual remains highly attractive during the whole season, another attracts few flies and two are intermediate. We obtained similar results in the 1985 season in our study herd where 75% of the flies were continually concentrated on less than 25% of the heifers.

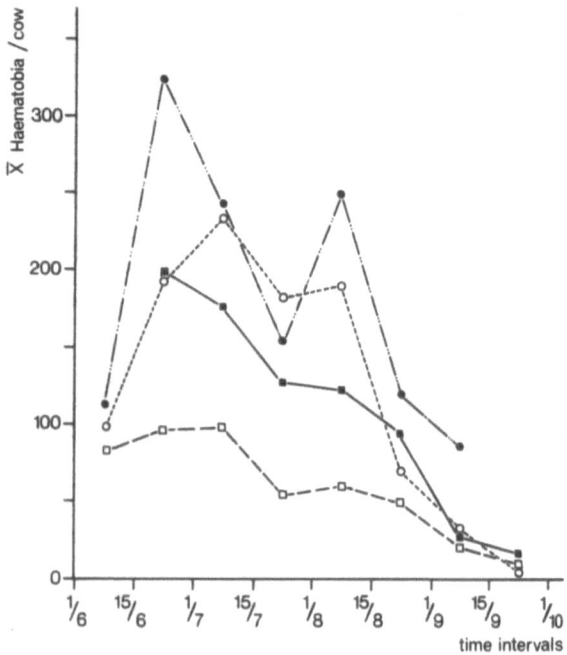

Fig. 1. Mean numbers of *Haematobia irritans* per 2 weeks on 4 individual cows. Data modified from Hammer (1941).

The remainder of this paper will describe some preliminary results obtained in the 1986 season where we concentrated on recording individual differences in fly pestation and made a start on elucidating the causality of these differences.

Figure 2 left gives the correlation between the total number of biting flies plotted against the total number of *Hydrotaea irritans* (the primary suspected vector of summer mastitis) for each individual in our K test herd. Not only do clear differences emerge between individuals with respect to attraction for flies but there appears to be a good correlation (r^2 = 0.92) between the number of biting flies and *H. irritans* ($p \ll 0.002$). In their totality, the correlation co-efficients for all four herds studied confirm this.

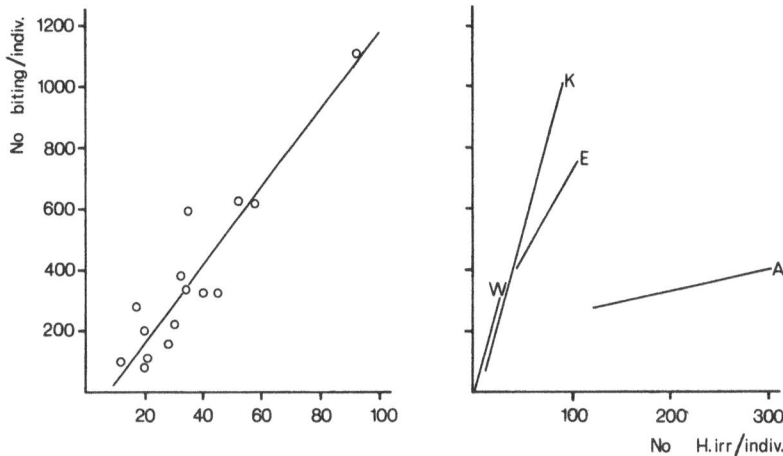

Fig. 2. Left: Correlation between the number of biting flies and *H. irritans* on each individual in the K test herd. Right: Regression lines for this correlation for all 4 herds observed.

Asking the question why some individuals are more attractive to flies than others is tantamount to determining the stimulus set used by the fly in selecting its host. Some of the variables involved have been discussed above. Other stimuli could well involve colour, pattern, temperature. Furthermore, earlier experiments showed that odour emanating from cattle can attract *H. irritans* (Thomas, 1983; Thomas *et al.*, 1985). As these host odours function in interspecific communication and, moreover, may result in deleterious consequences on the fitness of the individual producing them, they can be classified as kairomones.

To determine whether kairomones also contribute to differential risk between individual hosts, attraction tests were carried out in a wind-tunnel using single flies (for method see Thomas, 1983). The odour producing substrates tested were urine and washes from individual heifers. The washes were made both with ether and water (one on each side of the animal) to ensure removal of fat soluble and water soluble substances respectively. Two hundred and fifty ml. of solvent was applied to ~ 1 m² of the flank surface. The herd selected for this experiment was the A test herd which consisted of heifers of the dutch Red-White MRY breed.

To eliminate differences arising from other stimuli the method selected was to chose pairs of individuals which differed considerably in fly load but which were balanced in all other respects (*i.e.* hairiness, colour, marking pattern, age, pregnancy status). Table 2 gives the selected pairs and the predicted qualitative differences in attractiveness that would be expected in the wind-tunnel tests (*i.e.*, relative numbers of flies attracted to the odour source) if odour plays a role in an individual's attractiveness to flies.

TABLE 2. Differences in fly load between the selected pairs.

| | Selected pairs | | | | |
	70/60	49/59	106/105	108/109	110/113
Colour	red/white	red/white	red/white	red/white	red/white
% surface	90/10	25/75	40/60	35/65	10/90
Pregnant	+/+	+/+	−/−	−/−	−/−
H. irritans	220/29	270/117	150/69	175/76	140/116
Biting flies	243/105	325/118	292/116	187/40	126/76
Total	463/134	595/235	442/235	362/116	266/192
Predicted difference	70>60	49>59	106>105	108>109	110>113

Unlike the case in Tsetse flies (Owaga, 1985) no indication at all was found that urine attracts flies to the odour source in a wind-tunnel. The same may be said for the fat soluble wash, again not one fly reached the odour source in the wind-tunnel.

As far as the water wash was concerned however, 30% of the tested flies reached the odour source. This indicates that volatiles were present which attract *H. irritans*. Moreover, as can be seen in Table 3, the relative attractiveness of the odour deriving from the water washes fitted the predicted differences exactly.

TABLE 3. Relative attractiveness of the water washes in the wind-tunnel with respect to the predicted efficacy. (The number of flies tested/wash varied between 5—9).

Prediction	70>60	49>59	106>105	108>109	110>113
% flies reaching source	66.7/40	37.5/0	25/0	40/0	43/33.3

Sign test, p < 0.05.

In conclusion we may state that one of the causal factors underlying differences in attractiveness between heifers is one or more water soluble, volatile substances produced in or on the outer surface of the individual. Thus, differential risk between heifers in contracting summer mastitis is at least partly due to individual differences in host kairomone. The next step will be to carry out chemical analysis in order to identify the specific substances involved.

ACKNOWLEDGEMENTS

We wish to thank the National Animal Health Committee, the Hague and the Central Veterinary Institute for supporting the work and Mr. Muller for allowing us to use the facilities at Averheino Experimental Farm.

REFERENCES

Annual report Danish Pest Infestation Laboratory, 1984 (1985), DK-2800, Lyngby, Denmark.

Bock, R. 1980. Nachweis von *C. pyogenes* in Tonsillen und Lymphknoten von gesunden Kälbern und Jungrindern und dessen Bedeutung für das Auftreten der Sommermastitis, Vet. med. Diss. Hannover.

Bramley, A.J., Leaver, J.D., Kingwill, R.G. and Simpkin, D.L. 1977. *Corynebacterium pyogenes* mastitis among heifer calves. Vet. Rec., **100**, 464-465.

Bramley, A.J., Hillerton, J.E., Higgs, T.M. and Hogben, E.M. 1985. The carriage of summer mastitis pathogens by muscid flies. Br. Vet. J., **41**, 618-627.

Bjorn, H., Nansen, P., Hansen, J.W. and Nielsen, S. Achim. 1985. Sommermastitis. Forekomst på searlige graesningslokaliteter i Jylland. in "Initiativet Sommermastitits", (Report to the Danish Agricultural and Veterinary Research Council, Copenhagen.) ed. P. Nansen.

Dommerholt, G.J.G. Acute zomermastitis (zomerwrang): een gecompliceerd probleem, referaat C.H.L.S. Dronten, Gezondheidsdienst voor Dieren in Overijssel te Zwolle, October 1985.

Draper, N.R. and Smith, H. 1966. Applied Regression Analysis. John Wiley & Sons.

Egan, J. 1985. Evidence of *Corynebacterium pyogenes* as a secondary pathogen in mastitis in lactating cows. Kiel. Milch. Forschung., **37**, 585-588.

Everz, K.E. and Linge, F. 1979. Investigation of the incidence of heifer mastitis on Gotland. Publication No. 98 from the Swedish Association for Livestock Breeding and Production, 23-32. (In Swedish).

Francis, P.G., Wilesmith, J.W. and Wilson, C.D. 1986. Observations on the incidence of clinical bovine mastitis in non-lactating cows in England and Wales. Vet. Rec., **118**, 549-552.

Franke, V., Tolle, A., Reichmuth, J. and Beimgraben, J. 1983. Proc. Seminar of Heifer Mastitis, Stockholm - Helsinki, Swedish Association for Livestock and Production, Eskilstuna, Sweden.

Hammer, O. 1941. Biological and ecological investigations on flies associated with pastured cattle and their excrement. Vidensk. Medd. Dansk. Naturh. Foren., **105**, 141-393.

Hansen, J. and Nielsen, S.A. 1983. Summer mastitis. Proc. Heifer Mastitis Symp., Stockholm-Helsinki, Svensk Husdjursskotsel.

Hartigan, P.J. 1980. Fertility management in the dairy herd; the need to control bacterial contamination of the environment. Ir. Vet. J. **34**, 43-48.

Heidrich, H.J., Fiebiger, E., Utpott, J. 1964. Untersuchung uber die Pyogenes-Mastitis des Rindes mit besonderer Berucksichtigung der Fermenttherapie. I Mitt., Allgemeine Feststellung. BMTW, **77**, 234-236.

Hillerton, J.E., Bramley, A.J. and Watson, C.A. 1987. The epidemiology of summer mastitis; a survey of clinical cases. Br. Vet. J., (in press).

Jonsson, P. Olsson, S.O., Holmberg, O. and Funke, H. 1986. Heifer mastitis in Sweden during a three year period (1982 - 1985). Proceedings, XV Nordic Veterinary Congress, Stockholm, pp. 367-370. (In Swedish).

Klastrup, O. 1979. Definition of heifer mastitis. Publication No. 98 from the Swedish Association for Livestock Breeding and Production, 7-8. (In Swedish).

Knoef, J. Onderzoek naar de achtergronden van zomerwrang bij jongvee in Overijssel, referaat R.H.L.S. Deventer, Gezondheidsdienst voor Dieren in Overijssel te Zwolle, December 1981.

Lie, O. 1985. Genetic approach to mastitis control. Kiel. Milch. Forschung., 37, 487-488.

Lovell, R. 1943. The source of *Corynebacterium pyogenes* infections. Vet. Rec. 55, 99-100.

M.A.F.F. 1975-1985. Veterinary Investigation Diagnosis Analysis II. Central Veterinary Laboratory, Weybridge, U.K.

Marshall, A.B. 1981. Proc. of Seminar on mastitis control and herd management. Technical Bulletin No. 4, p. 81. National Institute for Research in Dairying, Reading. Hannah Research Institute, Scotland.

Meaney, W. and Egan, J. 1982. Mastitis — challenge from the environment. Proc. Moorepark Farmers Conf. May, 1982. 9-19.

Muller, M. 1977. Das Vorkommen der Pyogenesmastitis bei Jungrindern und Farsen unter Beruchsichtigung verschiedener Genanteile. Monat. Veterinaer., 32, 24-27.

Nielsen, Soren Achim. 1982. Ph. D. thesis, University of Aarhus, Denmark.

Nielsen, S. Achim. 1985. Attraktion af *Hydrotaea irritans* Fall. til gaessende kreaturer med saerligt henblik på betydingen af kvieharlegets farve samt patternes inbrydes position, pattefarve samt yverets beharing. In "Initiativet Sommermastitis", (Report to the Danish Agricultural and Veterinary Research Council, Copenhagen.) ed. P. Nansen.

Nielsen, S. Achim, Nielsen, B. Overgaard, Hansen, J.W., Nansen, P. and Olesen, J. 1983. Fourageringsaktivites hos *Hydrotaea irritans* i relation til klimaet. Report of the Danish Agricultural and Veterinary Research Council, Section 19, 239-245.

Niléhn, I. and Niléhn, P.O. 1953. Pasture mastitis in the county of Malmöhus in the summer of 1952. Publication for the members of the Swedish Veterinary Society, 5 (9), 101-102. (In Swedish).

Olesen, J.E., Nielsen, S. Achim, Hansen, J.W. and Nansen, P. 1985. The occurrence of summer mastitis in Jutland (Denmark) in relation to meteorological factors. Act. vet. scand., 26, 466-481.

O'Rourke, D.J., Chamings, R.J. and Booth, J.M. 1984. Summer mastitis surveys in England and Wales: 1978-1983. Vet. Rec., 115, 62-63.

Owaga, M.L.A. 1985. Observations on the efficacy of Buffalo urine as a potent olfactory attractant for *Glossina pallidipes* Austen. Insect Sci. Applic., 6, 561-566.

Pearson, J.K.L. 1951. Further experiments in the use of penicillin in the prevention of *C. pyogenes* infection of the non-lactating bovine udder, Vet. Rec., 68, 216-220.

Pettersson, K. 1980. Heifer mastitis within the areas of Gotland Milk-Recording Association and Kalmar AI and Milk-Recording Society — An inquiry. Swedish University of Agricultural Sciences, Department of Training of Agricultural and Horticultural Technologists, Alnarp. November. (In Swedish).

Saes, J.M.F. 1970. Voorkomen, pathogenese en bestrijding van *Corynebacterium pyogenes* mastitis (wrang) bij runderen in Limburg. Diss. R.U. te Utrecht.

Saes, J.M.F. 1971. Occurrence, pathogenesis and control of bovine *C. pyogenes*-mastitis (summer mastitis) in the province of Limburg, Tijdschr. Diergeneesk., 96, 1306-1317.

Saes, J.M.F. 1983. Heifer-mastitis, Tijdschr. Diergeneesk., 108, 554-555.

Schmoldt, P., Müller, H. and Motsch, T. 1974. Zur Pyogenesmastitis beim Jungrind, Mh. Vet.-Med., 29, 934-938.

Schwan, O. 1979. Heifer mastitis and dry cow mastitis. Thesis, Uppsala.

Schwan, O. and Holmberg, O. 1978/79. Heifer mastitis and dry cow mastitis: a bacteriological survey in Sweden. Vet. Microbiol. 3, 213-226.

Sieck, G. 1982. Arbeiten auf dem Gebiet der Pyogenes-Mastitis-Bekämpfung. Landeskontrollverband Schleswig-Holstein.

Sol, J. and Vardy, A. 1982. Effect of and length of protection offered by Cepravin Dry Cow® in the prevention of summer mastitis. Tijdschr. Diergeneesk., 107, 466-474.

Sol, J. 1983. Summer mastitis: Pathogenesis, losses, incidence and prevention. Tijdschr. Diergeneesk., **108**, 443-452.

Sol, J. 1984. Control Methods in summer mastitis: the importance of fly control. Proc. XIIIth World Congress on Diseases of Cattle, 236-242, Durban, S.A.

Sol, J., Vecht, U., Thomas, G. Summer mastitis: incidence, bacteriology, etiology, methods of prevention and entomological aspects. Proc. I.D.F. Seminar "Progress in the Control of Bovine Mastitis" pp. 21-24, May 1985, Kiel, F.R. Germany.

Sol, J., Vecht, U. and Thomas, G. 1985. Summer mastitis: incidence, bacteriology, aetiology. Methods of prevention and entomological aspects. Kiel. Milch. Forschung., **37**, 593-600.

Sorensen, G. Hoi. 1974. Studies on the aetiology and transmission of summer mastitis. Nord. Vet. Med., **26**, 122-133.

Sorensen, G.H. 1976. Studies on the occurrence of *Peptococcus indolicus* and *Corynebacterium pyogenes* in apparently healthy cattle. Act. Vet. Scand., **17**, 15-24.

Tarry, D.W. 1978. The headfly *Hydrotaea irritans* and summer mastitis infection. Vet. Rec., **102**, 91.

Thomas, G. 1983. Some preliminary investigations into the sensory and behavioural mechanisms of *Hydrotaea irritans*. Heifer Mastitis Seminar, Stockholm-Helsinki, Svensk. Husdjurrskotsel ek for.

Thomas, G., Schomaker, C.H., Been, T.H., van den Berg, M.J. and Prijs, H.J. 1985. Host finding and feeding in *Hydrotaea irritans* (Diptera: Muscidae): the role of chemical senses. Vet. Par., **18**, 209-221.

Tolle, A. and Reichmuth, J. 1985. Summer mastitis. Kiel. Milch. Forschung., **37**, 575-584.

Tolle, A., Reichmuth, J., Franke, V. and Beimgraben, J. 1985. Untersuchungen zur Pyogenes-Mastitis des Rindes. Kiel. Milch. Forschung., **36**, 125-212.

Untermann, F. 1965. Zur Aetiologie der Pyogenesmastitis. D. T. W., **72**, 482-486.

Wass, K. 1986. Trial with vaccination against heifer mastitis. Swed. Vet. J., **38**, 239-243. (In Swedish).

Weitz, B. 1949. *C. pyogenes* infection in cattle with special reference to summer mastitis, Vet. Rec., **61**, 123-126.

Wennemar, C. 1974. Untersuchungen zur Pyogenes-Mastitis des Rindes unter Einbeziehung eines Vakzinationsversuches. Vet. med. Diss., Hannover.

Yeoman, G.H. and Warren, B.C. 1984. Summer mastitis. Br. Vet. J., **140**, 232-243.

DISCUSSION

A difficulty in the discussion following the session of epidemiology was the absence of a common definition of summer mastitis.

Hydrotaea irritans is recognized as the main vector but also other dipterans were mentioned which could play a role in the transmission of the disease *e.g.* by damaging the teats, which would in turn attract *H. irritans*. It was also suggested that individual animals could exert a different attractivity for flies, possibly by means of their chemo-physical constitution or their fly dislodging behaviour. This is a subject for further study.

Dutch figures show a higher incidence of summer mastitis in high-yield cattle (animals producing 4-5 gallon/day). It was speculated that nutritional stress could play a role in the pathogenesis. Data from the U.K. do not support this hypothesis: the risk of infection in one quarter of a particular animal appears to be independant of the infection status of the other quarters. The incidence of animals with two or more summer mastitis quarters is low: less than 15% of the affected positive cases. Management factors could also contribute to the incidence of summer mastitis: 50% of the cases in the U.K. occur on farms with poor hygienic conditions. Concerning the pregnancy status it appeared difficult to be definite whether this influences susceptibility or not, because of the varying distribution of pregnant and non-pregnant animals over the year, and different periods of exposure to infection. Also the stage of pregnancy could play a role: Danish data suggest that pregnant animals are more susceptible to summer mastitis and that the risk for infection is higher in later stages as opposed to early pregnancy.

Depending on the individual disciplines of various researchers opinions were different as to what definition of summer mastitis would generally be acceptable. Clinicians tended to a definition on clinical signs, entomologists pressed the importance of fly transmission and the season, the bacteriologists favoured the bacteriological confirmation of a tentative clinical diagnosis. An important idea seems to define summer mastitis not so much on a specific bacteriological constitution or mode of transmission, but on a common prognosis and therapy. Important in this context was the observed close correlation in the Netherlands between prognosis and the presence of anaerobic bacteria. It was generally agreed that the definition of summer mastitis should refer to dry cattle with acute clinical mastitis with an as yet undefined, complex bacterial etiology (but in which *C. pyogenes* and obligate anaerobic bacteria seem important). But, if possible a more specific definition would be preferable: in the first place for the individual farmer and his veterinarian but also to make internationally comparable epidemiological studies possible.

2. BACTERIOLOGY OF THE DISEASE

Chairmen M. Madsen & O. Holmberg

THE BACTERIOLOGY OF SUMMER MASTITIS

M. Madsen

Institute of Hygiene and Microbiology,
Royal Veterinary and Agricultural University of Copenhagen,
13 Bülowsvej, DK–1870 Copenhagen V, Denmark

ABSTRACT

The paper reviews the bacteriology of summer mastitis in cattle. Recent bacteriological investigations of summer mastitis secretions have proved that summer mastitis is to be regarded as a complex polybacterial disease, with *Corynebacterium pyogenes, Peptococcus indolicus*, a non-classified microaerophilic coccus (Stuart-Schwan coccus), *Fusobacterium necrophorum, Bacteroides melaninogenicus*, and *Streptococcus dysgalactiae* as the most frequently isolated organisms. A brief outline of each of these bacterial species is presented, and their pathogenic potential discussed. The possible reservoirs of summer mastitis bacteria are listed, and finally the limited knowledge of synergistic bacterial interactions in the pathogenesis of summer mastitis is presented.

INTRODUCTION

Summer mastitis is cattle has been reported to occur in a number of European countries. Similar cases have been reported from Japan (Shimizu *et al.*, 1975; Shinjo *et al.*, 1976) and Australia (Slee and McOrist, 1985). The disease seems to be of most importance in Northern Europe, *e.g.* Holland, Germany, the UK, Sweden, and Denmark (Sorensen, 1979; Marshall, 1981), where it has been known for about a century (Glage, 1908). In Denmark, summer mastitis was reported for the first time in 1910 (Langhorn, 1910; Schmidt, 1910).

On clinical grounds, summer mastitis may be defined as covering cases of clinical mastitis occurring in non-lactating cattle, predominantly during the summer months. The syndrome is characterized by an acute suppurative mastitis, the secretion being thick, creamy and foul-smelling. Severe systemic reactions frequently occur (Sorensen, 1979; Marshall, 1981).

Although summer mastitis is a disease of very variable incidence from year to year and from farm to farm, the well defined seasonal incidence restricted to the summer months July, August, and September has repeatedly led to the suggestion of insects being involved in the transmission of the disease (Karmann, 1928; Bahr, 1952; Sorensen, 1974a, 1979; Hillerton *et al.*, 1983; Madsen, 1985).

Despite the fact that summer mastitis is also known as *Corynebacterium pyogenes* mastitis (Bramley *et al.*, 1977), it should be noted that the isolation of *C. pyogenes* is not a prerequisite to classification as summer mastitis. Although the prevalence of *C. pyogenes* in summer mastitis secretions is much higher than in mastitis secretions of lactating cattle (Schmidt Madsen *et al.*, 1974), the application of adequate procedures for the culturing of more fastidious microorganisms has revealed that most cases of summer mastitis yield mixed infections with at least five, or possibly more, bacterial species predominating. At present, it is difficult to define summer mastitis in exact bacteriological terms.

BACTERIOLOGICAL COMPOSITION OF SUMMER MASTITIS SECRETIONS

For a very long period *C. pyogenes* was considered the sole causal agent of summer mastitis. At the turn of the century the organism was isolated from mastitis secretions of lactating cattle (Glage, 1903) and a few years later suggested as the cause of summer mastitis (Glage, 1908).

Using anaerobic culture methods it was demonstrated that an anaerobe, *Peptococcus indolicus*, could be recovered regularly together with *C. pyogenes* from cases of bovine mastitis (Jorgensen, 1937). Applying similar techniques to samples from clinical summer mastitis, Stuart *et al.* (1951) demonstrated that about 90% of such samples yielded mixed bacterial cultures. They considered four bacterial species to be of particular note, namely *C. pyogenes, P. indolicus, Streptococcus dysgalactiae,* and a non-classifiable, Gram-positive microaerophilic coccus. This latter organism still remains to be named and properly classified in the present taxonomic system, but has tentatively been given the name "Stuart-Schwan coccus" (Sorensen, 1980).

TABLE 1   Frequency (%) of isolation of bacteria from field cases of summer mastitis after aerobic and anaerobic culture.

Organism	Ref. 1 (N=249)	Ref. 2 (N=22)	Ref. 3* (N=200)	Ref. 4 (N=88)	Ref. 5 (N=96)	Ref. 6 (N=168)
Cp	73	100	40	89	59	72
Pi	85	100	39	69	58	87
Ss	74	96	24	–	24	83
Fn	–	68	–	30	17	51
Bm	–	81	–	37	10	35
Sd	17	–	39	40	17	37

Cp = *Corynebacterium pyogenes*   Ref. 1 = Sorensen, 1974a
Pi = *Peptococcus indolicus*   Ref. 2 = Sorensen, 1978a
Ss = Stuart-Schwan coccus   Ref. 3 = Schwan and Holmberg, 1978/79
Fn = *Fusobacterium necrophorum*   Ref. 4 = Tolle *et al.*, 1983
Bm = *Bacteroides melaninogenicus*   Ref. 5 = Madsen, 1985
Sd = *Streptococcus dysgalactiae*   Ref. 6 = Madsen, *et al.*, 1985.
* = Investigated samples comprise secretions from heifer and dry cow mastitis collected during a one-year period.

Despite these observations, the view of summer mastitis as a monobacterial infection caused by *C. pyogens* was supported by several workers until the 1970's (Saes, 1971; Horsch *et al.*, 1974). During the last two decades, however, evidence of an increasing importance of obligate anaerobes in bovine mastitis has accumulated (Fiévez, 1965; Cornelisse *et al.*, 1970; Weber *et al.*, 1977; Aalbaek, 1978; Du Preez *et al.*, 1981; Shinjo, 1983). Two members of the family Bacteroidaceae, *Fusobacterium necrophorum* and *Bacteroides melaninogenicus*, have been regularly shown to occur in summer mastitis secretions (Sorensen, 1978a; Tolle *et al.*, 1983; Madsen, 1985; Madsen *et al.*, 1985).

In Table 1, the frequency of isolation of bacteria from summer mastitis secretions have been compiled from various authors. Although the results may not be directly comparable due to improvements in cultural techniques during the period, the data are at least uniform with regard to the bacterial complexity. According to the cited authors, summer mastitis secretions yield mixed cultures in approximately 90% of the cases. The combination of bacterial species in samples seems to vary somewhat between authors, but a very close relationship exists between *C. pyogenes, P. indolicus* and the Stuart-Schwan coccus. In ref. 6, the most common bacterial combination was *C. pyogenes, P. indolicus* and the Stuart-Schwan coccus mixed with *F. necrophorum* and/or *B. melaninogenicus* and/or *Str. dysgalactiae*, found in 64.5% of cases. In order to complete this rather confusing bacteriological picture of summer mastitis, mention should be given to the fact that occasionally other bacterial species, *e.g.* staphylococci, micrococci, streptococci, and *E. coli* have also been isolated from clinical cases of summer mastitis.

Experimental infections with summer mastitis have not been successful with pure cultures of *C. pyogenes*, whereas infusion of mixed cultures containing *C. pyogenes* and *P. indolicus* regularly results in the development of typical summer mastitis cases (Sorensen, 1972a). Similar results have been obtained by experimental infections with mixtures of *C. pyogenes, P. indolicus* and Stuart-Schwan coccus (Sorensen, 1972a; Schwan, 1979a) or with mixtures of *C. pyogenes, P. indolicus*, the Stuart-Schwan coccus and *Str. dysgalactiae* (Stuart *et al.*, 1951).

THE BACTERIAL SPECIES

Corynebacterium (s. Actinomyces) pyogenes

Taxonomically *C. pyogenes* has now been transferred to the genus *Actinomyces*, and should thus be named *Actinomyces pyogenes* (Anon., 1982). To avoid confusion, however, the name *C. pyogenes* is maintained throughout this paper.

C. pyogenes has been recovered from a wide range of pyogenic infections in cattle and swine (Sorensen, 1974a, 1974b, 1978b, 1979; Hartwigk, 1980). Isolated cases of human infections have been reported (Norenberg *et al.*, 1978; Lipton and Isalska, 1983). The pathogenic property of the organism is mainly ascribed to production of a thermolabile, necrotic hemolysin (Lovell, 1937). As to the biochemical and serological reactions of *C. pyogenes*, reference is made to Sorensen (1974b) and Hartwigk (1980).

C. pyogenes is widely distributed in apparently healthy cattle and swine. The preferred habitats of the organism include mucosal surfaces of the respiratory and reproductive tracts (Skovgaard, 1968; Sorensen, 1974a, 1976, 1978b).

Peptococcus indolicus

The organism was originally described under the name of *Micrococcus indolicus*, an anaerobic coccus isolated from bovine thelitis, galactophoritis (Christiansen, 1934) and mastitis (Jorgensen, 1937). Similar organisms isolated from mastitis secretions have been described as *Peptococcus asaccharolyticus* (Fiévez, 1965) and *Peptostreptococcus indolicus* (Cornelisse *et al.*, 1970). However, the name *Peptococcus indolicus* is presently accepted (Sorensen, 1974c), although recently a transfer to the genus Peptostreptococcus has been suggested (Ezaki *et al.*, 1983).

P. indolicus has so far not been isolated as the sole causal agent of pathological conditions in animals. In most cases it is isolated together with *C. pyogenes*, with which it seems to be a natural co-habitant, both in suppurative lesions and in clinically healthy animals (Sorensen, 1973, 1976, 1978b). A single case of human infection has been reported (Bourgault and Rosenblatt, 1979). *P. indolicus* is not hemolytic, although hemolysin-forming strains have been demonstrated (Sorensen, 1975). The principal pathogenic factor of *P. indolicus* seems to be a clotting factor, pepto-coagulase (Switalski *et al.*, 1978). Antigenic analyses have revealed the existence of six distinct serotypes, designated A–F, of which type B and C are most frequently isolated from summer mastitis secretions (Sorensen, 1973; Smyth *et al.*, 1980; Madsen *et al.*, 1985). Biochemical and enzymatic reactions have been described by Sorensen (1973) and Schwan (1979b). Of particular note is the production of indole and H_2S, which contribute to the foul smell of summer mastitis secretions.

The Stuart-Schwan coccus

At present the taxonomic position of this organism is uncertain. It was isolated for the first time from summer mastitis secretions in 1951 by Stuart *et al.* and described as "a microaerophilic coccus". The frequent occurrence in summer mastitis secretions (Table 1) indicates some kind of contribution to the pathogenesis, but its role is so far obscure. The Stuart-Schwan coccus seems to be a natural co-habitant with *C. pyogenes* and *P. indolicus*.

The biochemical and enzymatic reactions of the organism indicate that the investigated strains probably represent one species (Stuart, *et al.*, 1951; Sorensen, 1974a; Schwan, 1979a; Schwan *et al.*, 1979; Madsen, 1985; Slee, 1985). It might contribute to the spreading of infection due to the production of hyaluronidase (Sorensen, 1974a).

Bacteroidaceae

The family Bacteroidaceae comprises a large group of Gram negative, anaerobic rods, of which several are important pathogens in man and animals (Aalbaek, 1973; Berg and Loan, 1975; Chirino-Trejo and Prescott, 1983). Two species within this family are commonly encountered in summer mastitis secretions (Sorensen, 1978a; Tolle *et al.*, 1983; Madsen, 1985).

Bacteroides melaninogenicus is typically recovered from mixed human and animal infections (Fiévez, 1965; Biberstein *et al.*, 1968; Berg and Loan, 1975; Ingham *et al.*, 1975). Its natural habitat is seemingly the tonsils and the mucosal surfaces of the digestive tract (Heinrich *et al.*, 1959; LaLiberté and Mayrand, 1983).

Fusobacterium necrophorum is frequently isolated from a range of pathological conditions in ruminants and swine (Fiévez, 1963; Simon and Stovell, 1969; Berg and Loan, 1975; Langworth, 1977; Aalbaek, 1978; McGillivery and Nicholls, 1984). The natural reservoir of the organism is the oral cavity and the alimentary tract; in addition, the organism has been isolated from soil samples (Langworth, 1977). On serological and morphological grounds. *F. necrophorum* can be subdivided into two biotypes, A and B. This subdivision seems to correspond to differences in organ specificity; thus, strains recovered from mastitis samples can be classified as type B (Aalbaek, 1971, 1978; Madsen *et al.*, 1985), whereas biotypes involved in bovine liver abscesses belong to type A (Shinjo, 1983).

A wide spectrum of virulence factors have been described within the genera *Bacteroides* and *Fusobacterium* (Kasper and Finegold, 1979), which may be of importance in the pathogenesis of summer mastitis.

Streptococcus dysgalactiae

Str. dysgalactiae is a well-known mastitogen, serologically classified as group C streptococci. In relation to summer mastitis, the prevalence seems to vary between countries (Table 1). In contrast to the above-mentioned bacterial species, *Str. dysgalactiae* is recovered as a monoculture from summer mastitis sample more frequently, although it is also commonly encountered in mixed infections, (Madsen, *et al.*, 1985).

RESERVOIRS AND TRANSMISSION OF SUMMER MASTITIS BACTERIA

The bacterial species involved in summer mastitis seem to be well adapted to cattle and their environment, which is reflected in the repeated recovery of the organisms from tonsils, skin, mucous membranes, etc. in apparently healthy animals (Francis, 1941; Grupe, 1963; Sorensen, 1974a, 1976, 1978b; Nattermann and Horsch, 1977; Bock, 1980). In addition, the organisms have been demonstrated to be associated with suppurative conditions at numerous sites in cattle, *e.g.* abscesses, pneumonia, foul of the foot, metritis, and mastitis (Sorensen, 1974a; Hartwigk, 1980; Marshall, 1981). It has been demonstrated that the sporadic cases of Corynebacterium mastitis in stabled cattle yield mixed cultures similar to summer mastitis secretions, although the frequency of Bacteroidaceae may be higher in summer mastitis (Madsen, 1985; Nansen, 1985).

Thus, the main reservoir of summer mastitis bacteria can be considered to be associated with cattle themselves. On pastures, cattle are visited by a number of sucking and biting insects, of which the sheep headfly, *Hydrotaea irritans*, is the most numerous (Bahr, 1952; Marshall, 1981; Madsen, 1985; Nansen, 1985). Bacteriological investigations of symbovine dipteran species have revealed that the sucking species *Hydrotaea irritans*, and to some degree *Musca autumnalis* and *Morellia* spp., actually carry summer mastitis pathogens, whereas these are very rarely isolated from biting, haematophageous species (Sorensen, 1974a; Michael, 1983; Nansen, 1985; Bramley *et al.*, 1985). The infection of *H. irritans*, as regards *C. pyogenes* and *P. indolicus*, has been demonstrated to persist for at least seven days and possibly longer (Madsen, 1985).

The transmission of summer mastitis bacteria to healthy, grazing cattle may thus take place when sucking symbovine flies, in particular *H. irritans*, become infected by feeding on contaminated animals and hereafter visit the teats of healthy animals. This view is supported by the fact that flies caught in early summer, *i.e.* June and July, are usually found to be bacteriologically sterile, whereas the bacterial contamination of flies as well as healthy cattle teats culminates in the first week of August. Actual figures amount to approximately 10% infected *H. irritans* and 80% contaminated healthy teats at this time (Nansen, 1985). At this point it should be stressed that animals attacked by summer mastitis remain infected for weeks (Schwan, 1980; Schwan and Smyth, 1980; Madsen, 1985) despite treatment, and thus constitute an important reservoir of infection to pastured cattle if not removed.

CONCLUDING REMARKS ON THE BACTERIAL CONTRIBUTION OF THE PATHOGENESIS OF SUMMER MASTITIS

It has been proposed that summer mastitis develops as an activation of latent, subclinical udder infections (Nattermann and Horsch, 1977). However, bacteriological examinations of juvenile udder secretions have not revealed any bacterial species associated with summer mastitis (Ohm, 1958; Sorensen, 1979; Madsen, 1985).

The infection route of summer mastitis may thus be considered to take place via the teat canal, where predisposing factors such as breed, pregnancy status, teat injuries, etc. may play an important role. With regard to the bacterial species involved, an impressive spectrum of virulence factors have been demonstrated within these species, as compiled in Table 2.

TABLE 2. Potential virulence factors produced by bacterial species commonly encountered in summer mastitis secretions.

Bacterium	Factor
C. pyogenes	Hemolysin
	Sphingomyelinase
	Protease
	Neuraminase
	Pili
P. indolicus	Peptocoagulase
	Deoxyribonuclease
Stuart-Schwan coccus	Hyaluronidase
	Deoxyribonuclease
	Chondroitin sulphatase
F. necrophorum	Leucocidin
	Hemolysin
	Necrogenic toxin
B. melaninogenicus	Collagenase
	Ig-protease
	Proteases
	Capsular polysaccharide
	Pili

(Data compiled from Müller, 1973; Yanagawa and Honda, 1976; Kasper and Finegold, 1979; Schwan, 1979a; Takeuchi et al., 1979; Fujimura and Nakamura, 1981; Carlsson et al., 1984; Emery et al., 1984).

Although typical, clinical summer mastitis can be reproduced by the infusion of only two of these species (C. pyogenes and P. indolicus) (Sorensen, 1972a), it appears logical that the other frequently isolated bacteria contribute either in the establishment of the infection or by aggravating the clinical symptoms. Synergistic interactions between C. pyogenes and Bacteroidaceae have been reported to be of etiological significance in closely related polybacterial syndromes (Roberts, 1967a, 1967b; Roberts et al., 1968; Kaufman et al., 1972; Brook et al., 1984), and similar interactions may be of importance in summer mastitis infection. Studies by Sorensen (1980) have demonstrated a stimulating effect of P. indolicus and Stuart-Schwan cocci on the toxin production of C. pyogenes in co-cultures, but otherwise the present knowledge of other interactions and potentiating effects in the complex microbial ecosystem of summer mastitis is very limited. In the light of the hitherto disappointing results of the immunoprophylaxis of summer mastitis (Sorensen, 1972b: Cameron and Fuls, 1977), future research into the effects of virulence factors, especially with regard to adhesion factors (Lee et al., 1983) should be given emphasis.

HEIFER MASTITIS IN SWEDEN DURING A 3 YEARS PERIOD (1982–1985). BACTERIOLOGICAL FINDINGS IN UDDER SECRETION FROM CLINICAL AND SUBCLINICAL CASES

P. Jonsson*, **, S.–O. Olsson***, O. Holmberg*, ****, H. Funke*** and A.–S. Olofson*

*National Veterinary Institute, S–750 07 Uppsala, Sweden.
**Present address: Ewos AB, Box 618, S–151 27 Södertälje, Sweden.
***Swedish Association for Livestock Breeding and Production,
Animal Health Department, Eskilstuna, Sweden.
****Swedish University of Agricultural Sciences, Department of Veterinary Microbiology,
Section of Clinical Microbiology, Uppsala, Sweden.

ABSTRACT

Milk samples from 1487 heifers with symptoms of clinical mastitis and secretions from 351 clinically healthy heifers were bacteriologically investigated. *Streptococcus dysgalactiae, Streptococcus uberis, Staphylococcus aureus, Escherichia coli* and *Actinomyces (Corynebacterium) pyogenes* were the most frequently isolated bacterial species of clinical heifer mastitis. These bacteria, *Peptostreptococcus indolicus*, Stuart-Schwan cocci and strict anaerobic bacteria were often isolated as mixed infections. The frequency of clinical cases of heifer mastitis is largest in July-September but the distribution between different bacterial species is almost the same at different times of the year. Most of the cases were seen during the first week post-partum. Coagulase-negative staphylococci were the dominating bacteria in clinically healthy heifers.

INTRODUCTION

In earlier Swedish investigations (Everz and Linge, 1975; Schwan, 1979) *Corynebacterium (Actinomyces) pyogenes* were among the most frequently isolated bacteria but they occurred most often as mixed infections with *Peptococcus (Peptostreptococcus) indolicus* and a microaerophilic coccus (Stuart-Schwan coccus) in the same udder quarter. *Streptococcus dysgalactiae* were also often found as well as *Streptococcus uberis* and *Staphylococcus aureus.*

The cited investigations were based on relatively few clinical cases concentrated mainly on the island of Gotland. Therefore, a wider bacteriological investigation of the etiology of mastitis in heifers was undertaken between 1982–1985. This study also included bacteriological investigation of secretions from clinically healthy heifers. Preliminary results are presented in this report.

MATERIALS AND METHODS

The definition of heifer mastitis proposed at a nordic seminar, 1978, has been used in this study (Olsson *et al.*, 1986). This means that the investigation covers all cases of mastitis in heifers according to the definition, including "*A. pyogenes* — anaerobe complex" (summer mastitis) cases.

Practicing veterinarians sent milk samples from affected quarters of all heifers reported with mastitis from eight representative areas covering the different geographic regions and biotopes of Sweden. The number per month of all investigated heifers (1487) with symptoms of clinical mastitis are presented in Table 1. The secretions were taken in 10 ml plastic tubes (A/S Nunc, Roskilde, Denmark) after cleaning the teat with alcohol (70%). A small amount (1–2 ml) of the secretion was transfered into an oxygen free, glass ampule (approximately 4 ml) by using a syringe (5 ml) and needle.

TABLE 1.   Monthly numbers and percentages of heifers with clinical mastitis in 8 areas during 1982–1985

	Jan	Febr	March	April	May	June	July	Aug	Sept	Oct	Nov	Dec	Total number of cases
1982/83													
Number	20	29	12	9	3	7	20	85	90	50	69	32	426
Percentage	4.7	6.8	2.8	2.1	0.7	1.6	4.7	20.9	21.1	11.7	16.2	7.5	
1983/84													
Number	27	18	13	10	16	5	35	157	104	80	74	33	572
Percentage	4.7	3.1	2.3	1.7	2.8	0.9	6.1	27.4	18.2	14.0	12.9	5.8	
1984/85													
Number	33	26	12	10	4	1	23	111	93	85	60	31	489
Percentage	6.7	5.3	2.5	2.0	0.8	0.2	4.7	22.7	19.0	17.4	12.3	6.3	
Total													
Number	80	73	37	29	23	13	78	353	287	215	203	96	1487
Percentage	5.4	4.9	2.5	2.0	1.5	0.9	5.2	23.7	19.3	14.5	13.7	6.5	

The bacteriological investigation was, with few exceptions, performed the day after sampling. The aerobic investigation was performed according to Klastrup and Schmidt Madsen (1974) while the anaerobic one was made according to the VPI Anaerobe Laboratory Manual (Holdeman et al., 1977).

For the investigation of secretions from clinically healthy heifers, samples were collected in the same way as for clinical cases. The samples were taken from all four quarters of heifers in the period 0–7 days post-partum in the countries of Gotland and Östergötland.

RESULTS AND DISCUSSION

The following aerobic bacteria, which are also commonly isolated from mastitis in lactating cows, were isolated from the investigated secretions from clinical mastitis cases in heifers: streptococci, 67.1%; staphylococci, 32.0%; and *Escherichia coli*, 17.1%. *Actinomyces pyogenes*, *Peptostreptococcus indolicus* and Stuart-Schwan cocci, all usually associated with summer mastitis in heifers, were isolated at low frequences: 13.4; 9.2; and 6.3% respectively. *Fusobacterium necrophorum*, *Bacterioides melaninogenicus* and other anaerobic bacteria were isolated at low frequences (Table 2). Previous investigations in many countries, including Sweden, (Everz and Linge, 1975; Schwan, 1979), have reported higher frequencies of infections caused by *A. pyogenes*. This bacterium was isolated in 59% of Danish cases (Madsen, 1985) and from West Germany (Franke, *et al.*, 1983) 89% was reported. However, in these investigations the definition of heifer mastitis was different from that used in the present study.

TABLE 2.   Distribution of different bacteria isolated from 1487 clinical cases of heifer mastitis.

	No. of isolates	%	% heifers yielding
Staphylococcus aureus	305	13.0	20.5
Coagulase-negative staphylococci	171	7.3	11.5
Streptococcus agalactiae	2	0.08	0.1
Streptococcus dysgalactiae	605	25.9	40.7
Streptococcus uberis	321	13.7	21.6
Other streptococci	70	3.0	4.7
Escherichia coli	254	10.9	17.1
Other coliform bacteria	26	1.1	1.7
Other aerobic bacteria	41	1.8	2.8
Actinomyces pyogenes	199	8.5	13.4
Stuart-Schwan cocci	94	4.0	6.3
Peptostreptococcus indolicus	137	5.9	9.2
Fusobacterium necrophorum *Fusobacterium* spp	63	2.7	4.4
Bacteroides melaninogenicus *Bacteroides* spp	17	0.7	1.1
Clostridum perfringens	14	0.6	0.9
Other anaerobic bacteria	18	0.8	1.2
Yeast	1	0.04	0.06
No. of bact. isolates	2338		

Table 3 shows the infection pattern of cases occuring pre-partum and on pasture from May to October. The incidences of *A. pyogenes*, Stuart-Schwan cocci, *Peptostreptococcus indolicus* and other anaerobic bacteria were higher than the incidences of these species in the complete material (Tables 2 and 3).

TABLE 3.   Bacteriological investigation of secretions from clinical cases of mastitis in pre-partum heifers, on pasture during May-October.

Bacteria	No of isolates	% heifers yielding
Staphylococcus aureus	26	10.6
Coagulase-negative staphylococci	31	12.7
Streptococcus agalactiae	1	0.4
Streptococcus dysgalactiae	98	40.0
Streptococcus uberis	39	15.9
Other streptococci	9	3.7
Escherichia coli	21	8.6
Other coliforms	3	1.2
Other aerobic bacteria	9	3.7
Actinomyces pyogenes	72	29.4
Stuart-Schwan cocci	35	14.3
Peptostreptococcus indolicus	60	24.5
Fusobacterium necrophorum	39	15.9
Bacteroides melaninogenicus	10	4.1
Other anaerobic bacteria	1	0.4
No. of heifers	**245**	

Table 4 shows the distribution of isolated bacteria within a quarter of a year from 1487 clinical cases of heifer mastitis. The frequency of cases is largest in July-September but the distribution between different bacterial species is about the same in different periods of the year.

In the present study most of the clinical cases of mastitis in heifers occured during the first week post-partum. According to Danish investigations (Hansen and Nielsen, 1983) the disease is more common in the last third of the pregnancy, but again the definition was different.

TABLE 4.   Distribution of isolated bacteria within a quarter of a year from 1487 clinical cases of heifer mastitis.

Bacteria	Jan-March I		April-June II		July-Sept III		Oct-Dec IV	
		%		%		%		%
Staphylococcus aureus	66	22.0	20	22.2	105	8.9	114	14.9
Coagulase-negative staphylococci	25	8.3	10	11.1	87	7.3	49	6.4
Streptococci	91	30.3	31	34.4	542	45.9	334	43.6
Coliform bacteria	39	13.0	14	15.6	125	10.6	102	13.3
Other aerobic bacteria	11	3.7	2	2.2	21	1.8	8	1.0
Actinomyces pyogenes	33	11.0	8	8.9	91	7.7	67	8.7
Stuart-Schwan cocci	9	3.0	1	1.1	58	4.9	26	3.4
Peptostreptococcus indolicus	14	4.7	4	4.4	82	6.9	37	4.8
Anaerobic bacteria	12	4.0	0	0	71	6.0	29	3.8
No. of isolated strains	300		90		1182		766	

TABLE 5.   Distribution of bacteria isolated from clinically healthy heifers in two Swedish areas.

Bacterial species	No. of isolates Gotland		Östergötland	
		%		%
Staphylococcus aureus	9	1.2	12	1.7
Coagulase-negative staphylococci	113	16.2	87	12.3
Streptococci	18	2.6	30	4.2
Coliform bacteria (*E. coli*)	5	0.7	9	1.3
Other aerobic bacteria	9	1.2	2	0.3
Actinomyces pyogenes	0	0	1	0.1
Stuart-Schwan cocci	0	0	1	0.1
Peptostreptococcus indolicus	0	0	1	0.1
No. of investigated samples	696		708	
No. of investigated heifers	174		177	

Table 5 shows the distribution of bacteria isolated from clinically healthy heifers 0–7 days post-partum. Most samples were bacteriologically negative. Coagulase-negative staphylococci were the most frequently isolated bacteria but also other species were found in low numbers. Our results agree with those of Daniel et al., 1986 in Canada and also with an investigation of pre-partum secretions from clinically healthy heifers collected for market (S.-O. Olsson and P. Jonsson, personal communication).

In conclusion, most cases of mastitis in heifers in the eight different areas in Sweden, were caused by Streptococci, Staphylococci and coliforms, the species usually associated with mastitis in lactating cows.

The incidences of A. pyogenes, Stuart-Schwan cocci, Peptostreptococcus indolicus and other anaerobic bacteria were relatively low. According to a preliminary study in which heifers were systemically treated with antibiotics for 3-5 days, approximately 80% of the udders were bacteriologically negative (after one and eight weeks) and clinically healthy (C. Tideström, P. Jonsson and G. Åström, to be published). The farmers are, therefore, advised to control the udder of the heifers very carefully, daily if possible, in order to facilitate an early treatment.

Subclinical mastitis in heifers caused by major pathogens seems to be rare. Coagulase-negative staphylococci were the most prominent species found (approximately 14% of the udder quarters).

ACKNOWLEDGEMENT

The Farmer's Research Council for Information and Development financially supported this work.

THE BACTERIOLOGICAL CONSTITUTION OF DUTCH SUMMER MASTITIS CASES

U. Vecht*, H.J. Wisselink*, J. Sol**, A.E.J.M. van den Bogaard***

*Central Veterinary Institute,
P.O. Box 65, 8200 AB Lelystad, The Netherlands.
**Animal Health Service, Zwolle, The Netherlands.
***University of Limburg, Maastricht, The Netherlands.

ABSTRACT

In 1984 and 1985, 51 udder secretions collected from heifers and dry cows suspected of having contracted summer mastitis were examined bacteriologically for the presence of facultative anaerobic and obligate anaerobic bacteria (OAB). The effect of therapy with Spiramycin in 1984 and Penicillin/Cloxacillin in 1985 was examined both bacteriologically and clinically.

Corynebacterium pyogenes was isolated in 35% of the cases. Other species which are also associated with mastitis such as *Peptococcus indolicus* and *Fusobacterium necrophorum* were isolated in 31% and 22% respectively. In 18%, OAB mostly in combination with other bacteria were isolated but the presence of *C. pyogenes* could not be demonstrated. These cases still showed symptoms typical for summer mastitis. The incidence of summer mastitis during the trial was low in the sample area: 0.30% in 1984 and 0.15% in 1985 compared to 10% in 1980. This might have caused these relatively low isolation rates.

Therapy with antibiotics had little effect on affected quarters when OAB, with or without *Corynebacterium pyogenes*, were involved. Systemic symptoms generally disappeared after treatment. Both therapy with Spiramycin/Colistine and Penicillin/Cloxacillin gave good results in suspected summer mastitis cases, but caused by facultative anaerobic bacteria. This emphasizes the need for a correct and rapid diagnosis as the prognosis is dependant on the presence c.q. absence of obligate anaerobic bacteria. It is subject to discussion whether *C. pyogenes* or OAB are more characteristic in the etiology of summer mastitis.

INTRODUCTION

At present a variety of bacterial species can be isolated from cases of acute mastitis in dry cattle, clinically typical for summer mastitis. Originally, this condition was solely referred to as *Corynebacterium pyogenes* mastitis (Glage, 1903; Poels, 1910). Later, more attention was given to the involvement of other bacteria. A number of species are often isolated from field cases such as *Peptococcus indolicus, Streptococcus dysgalactiae, Fusobacterium necrophorum* and *Bacteroides* spp. The role of non-sporulating, obligate anaerobic bacteria (OAB) has been a particular subject of research (Cornelissen, 1970; Sorensen, 1974a; Seno and Azuma, 1983; Greef et al. 1983).

This report deals with the bacteriological findings from cases of acute mastitis of heifers and dry cows in The Netherlands and their response to treatment with antibiotics.

MATERIALS AND METHODS

In the summers of 1984 and 1985 twin samples were collected from non-lactating heifers and cows, suspected of having contracted summer mastitis. Farms participating in this study were situated in an area with a high incidence of summer mastitis in the previous years (10% in 1980). (Sol et al., 1985). The teat was cleaned and disinfected with Sterilon[®] and the sample was taken using a disposable plastic syringe.

After expiration of all air from syringe and needle the sample was injected into a Port-a-cul vial[®] [1] and mailed to the laboratory. After arrival the samples were processed both aerobically and anaerobically. The latter by using an anaerobic glovebox (10% H_2, 80% CO_2, 10% N_2).

After five days of treatment the animals were again sampled and the samples processed as described.

THERAPY

Different therapies were applied in 1984 and 1985. In 1984, animals were treated with 10 g Spiramycine (Suanovil[®])[2] intramuscularly at day 1 and 3 and intramamillary with a combination of Spiramycine and Colistine (Mammivert[®])[2] daily. Affected quarters were stripped daily before therapy was administered.

In 1985, therapy consisted of intramuscular administration of 10 million U. Na penicillin and 6 million U. Procaine benzylpenicillin on day 1 and daily intramamillar application of cloxacillin (Orbenin[®] quick release)[3] for 5 days. Again, affected quarters were stripped before this treatment was applied.

BACTERIOLOGY

Smears were stained with Gram's method. The samples were processed for isolation of facultative anaerobic and microaerophilic organisms using 10% ox blood agar, Hauge-Edwards tryptose (H.E.T.) medium, 6% horse blood Columbia agar base and thioglycollate broth. Identification was according to the methods of Cowan and Steel (1974). In addition, the commercial identification systems API-Staph[®] and API Strep[®][4] were used.

Streptococci were also classified serologically according to Lancefield using a coagglutination test (Streptex[®])[5]. This test can identify A, B, C, D, F and G groups. Aspecific negative and group D strains were further tested with polysaccharide extraction procedures using Fuller extracts and commercial test sera[5].

For isolation of obligate anaerobic bacteria a modified Wensinck medium with and without anitbiotics (neomycin or kanamycin and vancomycin) Brain Heart Infusion

[1] Becton & Dickinsen Lab., Amersfoort.
[2] Rhone-Poulenc, Nederland B.V., Amstelveen.
[3] Beecham Farma B.V., Amstelveen.
[4] API Benelux 's-Hertogenbosch.
[5] Wellcome Reagents Ltd., Weesp.

(BHI) agar (supplemented) with 6% horse blood and BHI (supplemented) broth and thio-glycollate broth (supplemented) were used.

Plates were incubated in an anaerobic glove box at 37°C and checked for growth every 48 hrs for one week. Identification was carried out using standard anaerobic identification procedures (Holdeman, Cato & Moore, 1977) and with the API -20 A® test system[1]. (Pepto) coagulase production was assayed using a tube clotting test with bovine plasma.

The concentration of Spiramycin was measured in blood sera and udder secretions. The technique is based on measuring the zone of inhibition for Sarcina lutea (ATCC 9341) in a standardized medium (Milieu Agar No 5 Merck) and comparing the zone with a standard Spiramycin solution; the diameter of the zone is proportional to the logarithm of the concentration.

RESULTS

A. Identity and frequency of bacteria.

Of the 51 specimens collected from 48 cases, 49 yielded a positive culture. Both facultative anaerobic and obligate anaerobic bacteria (OAB) were isolated. The results are given in Table 1.

TABLE I.   Bacteriology of 51 secretions collected from 48 dry cattle during summer

	number	percentage
Number of secretions	51	
Sterile secretions	2	4
Combinations with C. pyogenes	18	35
Combinations with OAB, without C. pyogenes	9	18
Combinations with other bacteria	22	43

C. pyogenes could be isolated in only 18 specimens (35%). Mixtures of various species of obligate anaerobic bacteria, but without C. pyogenes, were cultured from 9 samples (18%). In 22 cases, other facultative anaerobic bacteria were isolated. Such cases are not to be considered as summer mastitis.

Up to 8 species could be isolated from one specimen. The range of obligate anaerobic bacteria only was 1—5. The range of facultative anaerobic bacteria 1—4. The identity of the bacterial species and their frequency of isolation are shown in Table 2.

[1] API Benelux 's-Hertogenbosch.

TABLE 2. Bacterial species isolated from 49 culture-positive mastitis secretions

Organism	Frequency of isolation	Percentage of positive cases
Facultative anaerobes		
Bacillus spp.	12	24
Corynebacterium pyogenes	18	37
Staphylococci (coagulase +ve)	3	6
Staphylococci (coagulase −ve, 7 species)	25	51
Streptococcus acidominimus	2	4
Streptococcus dysgalactiae	4	8
Streptococcus equisimilis	2	4
Streptococcus mitis	3	6
Streptococcus uberis	8	16
other streptococci	6	12
Enterococci	3	6
Escherichia coli	1	2
Candida spp.	1	2
Total	88	
Obligate anaerobes		
Bacteroides melaninogenicus	4	8
Bacteroides oralis	1	2
Fusobacterium necrophorum	11	22
Bifidobacterium bifidum	2	4
Clostridium perfringens	2	4
Clostridium sporogenes	3	6
Clostridium butyricum	1	2
Clostridium ramosum	1	2
Peptococcus indolicus	16	33
Streptococcus anaerobius	1	2
Total	42	

The most frequently isolated facultative anaerobic species, are *Corynebacterium pyogenes* (37%) and coagulase negative Staphylococci (51%), a wide variety of Streptococci was observed including species which are uncommon in bovine mastitis.

Of the obligate anaerobic species, *Fusobacterium necrophorum* and *Peptococcus indolicus* were found in percentages of 22% and 33% respectively, *Bacteroides* spp. in 10%. The *Clostridium* spp. could often only be isolated after incubation in fluid media such as thioglycollate broth, indicating that these were present in low numbers only.

B. Effect of therapy.

The effect of therapy with Spiramycin/Colistine (1984) on the various organisms is shown in Table 3.

TABLE 3.　　　Isolations of bacteria after treatment with Spiramycin/Colistine

days after treatment:	day 1	day 5
C. pyogenes	5	5
F. necrophorum	6	3
Bacteroides spp.	3	2
P. indolicus	5	5
mixtures with OAB and/or *C. pyogenes*	11	10
facultative anaerobic bacteria	13	2

It appears that despite treatment with Spiramycine/Colistine, obligate anaerobic bacteria and *C. pyogenes* are still viable in summer mastitis secretions, as opposed to facultative anaerobic bacteria which do not survive this treatment in the majority of the cases.

The effect of therapy with Penicillin/Cloxacillin (1985) on the various organisms is given in Table 4.

TABLE 4.　　　Isolations of bacteria after treatment with Penicillin/Cloxacillin

days after treatment:	day 1	day 5
C. pyogenes	5	2
F. necrophorum	2	1
Bacteroides spp.	1	0
P. indolicus	4	1
mixtures with OAB and/or *C. pyogenes*	6	2
facultative anaerobic bacteria	8	3

The effect of treatment with Penicillin/Cloxacillin, when examined bacteriologically, seems slightly better than the Spiramycin/Colistine treatment: *C. pyogenes* and OAB were not isolated from some secretions after 5 days of treatment. The number of total samples however, was very small.

Spiramycin concentrations in serum (n=23) measured after 5 days of treatment averaged 0.33 μg/ml (s.d. 0.16) and in udder secretions (n=21), 146 μg/ml (s.d. 245). Concentrations in sera were quite similar, in contrast to those in udder secretions with large variations. The average spiramycin concentration in udder secretions of mastitis cases caused by facultative anaerobic bacteria was lower (99 μg/ml) than that of cases complicated by obligate anaerobic bacteria (192 μg/ml).

DISCUSSION

An isolation rate of 35% for *C. pyogenes* in cases suspected of summer mastitis is relatively low according to results obtained by others (Sorensen, 1974a, 1978a; Tolle *et al.*, 1983). However, despite the fact that *P. indolicus* was the most common OAB isolated, an isolation rate of 33% is lower than in most other recent publications (Cornelisse *et al.*, 1970; Sorensen, 1974a and 1978a; Tolle *et al.*, 1983). As a matter of fact most authors isolated *P. indolicus* at an even greater frequency than *C. pyogenes* from summer mastitis secretions.

Several explanations can be given for these differences. During the survey periods the summer mastitis incidence was very low compared to previous years, probably because of preventive measures: the use of fly repellants (so called ear tags) on animals at risk and a low population density of the vector (flies) due to climatological conditions (relatively cold springs). Moreover samples were taken from dry cows and heifers, after the farmer had called his veterinary surgeon to a case of acute mastitis in the summer. Therefore, a relatively high number of specimens was not obtained from cows suffering from summer mastitis but from other types of mastitis which occur in dry cattle. It appears that apart from summer mastitis also other types of mastitis occur in dry cattle in the summer, which could lead to unjustified culling of animals.

Clinically there was no difference between infections by *C. pyogenes* combined with obligate anaerobic bacteria and infections by OAB only: these patients showed mostly general symptoms, lack of appetite, fever and a stiff gait, the affected quarter was hard and responded poorly to therapy. This raises the question of whether *C. pyogenes* is essential in the etiology of summer mastitis, and whether certain OAB, such as *P. indolicus, F. necrophorum* and *Bacteroides* spp. should be considered as primary or secondary pathogens. Tolle *et al.* (1983) reported that in 78% of cases which they had examined *C. pyogenes* was combined with obligate anaerobes, other combinations occurred in lower frequency.

If OAB are characteristic for summer mastitis it should be possible to make a rapid and reliable diagnosis by direct demonstration of the presence of their metabolic products in summer mastitis secretions. Volatile fatty acids are such products and gas chromatography is suitable for detecting these, as was shown for pus from swine abcesses (Van den Bogaard,

1983).

Therapy resulted in only limited success in cases where obligate anaerobic bacteria were involved: clinically, general health condition improved after therapy but the affected quarter was lost for further production. In vitro, despite treatment with antibiotics, bacteria could often be reisolated after 5 days. Spiramycin treatment did not result in any better cure *in vivo* or *in vitro* than the Penicillin/Cloxacillin therapy. When only facultative anaerobic bacteria were involved, both therapies were quite successful, not only measured bacteriologically but also clinically: in 19 out of the 23 cases the affected quarters also became normal. This emphasizes the importance of a rapid and reliable diagnosis as the prognosis for affected quarters differs, depending on the involvement of obligate anaerobic bacteria.

The relatively high incidence of cases with symptoms typical for summer mastitis (hard quarter, often with fever and/or typical secretum) with OAB, but without *C. pyogenes* 8/28 (29%) was remarkable. These quarters also responded poorly to therapy, as did "ordinary" cases of summer mastitis with *C. pyogenes*. It therefore becomes questionable whether summer mastitis can still be named the *C. pyogenes*/OAB complex (Tolle *et al.*, 1983). Du Preez *et al.* (1982) reported that OAB can cause considerable damage to the bovine udder in the absence of other organisms.

As summer mastitis was in the past only attributed to *C. pyogenes* (Glage, 1903; Poels, 1910) later to *C. pyogenes* and peptococci (Saes, 1970; Cornelissen, 1970; Sorensen, 1974a) still later to *C. pyogenes* with OAB, it now looks as if OAB alone or in combination with other bacteria but not necessarily with *C. pyogenes*, can cause this disease. Further studies are necessary to clarify this.

ACKNOWLEDGMENTS

The authors wish to thank Dr. J. Haagsma for technical assistance with the bacteriology of anaerobes and Dr. J.M.F. Nouws for making the facilities available to assess Spiramycin values. Without the cooperation of the veterinary practioners in the area of the Animal Health Service Institute in Overijssel this study would not have been possible. The financial support of the National Animal Health Committee is gratefully acknowledged.

GASCHROMATOGRAPHIC ANALYSIS OF SUMMER MASTITIS SECRETIONS FOR THE PRESUMPTIVE DIAGNOSIS OF INFECTIONS BY OBLIGATE ANAEROBIC BACTERIA

A.E. van den Bogaard*, U. Vecht**, J. Sol***

*Department of Medical Microbiology, University of Limburg,
P.O. Box 616, 6200 MD Maastricht, The Netherlands.
**Central Veterinary Institute, Lelystad, The Netherlands.
***Animal Health Service, Zwolle, The Netherlands.

ABSTRACT

Udder secretions sampled during the summer in 1984 and 1985 from mastitis quarters of 51 non-lactating heifers and dry cows were examined bacteriologically for the presence of (facultative) aerobic and obligate anaerobic bacteria (OAB) and by gas liquid chromatography (GLC) in order to detect volatile fatty acids (VFA), metabolic endproducts of OAB. Forty-nine samples yielded positive cultures and in 20 cases these were mixtures of (facultative) aerobes and OAB. Only 2 specimens appeared to be sterile and from one specimen only OAB were cultured. In most specimens (19/21) which yielded OAB after culturing, VFA (C_3-C_6) could be detected by GLC. A specific pretreatment method had to be developed for GLC-analysis of udder secretions to avoid interfering peaks on the chromatogram and to prevent poisoning of the GLC-column. Two false negatives and one false positive were noted. Detection of VFA by GLC-analysis in summer mastitis secretions appeared to be a useful technique for evaluating the importance and association of OAB with summer mastitis. Because samples can be easily collected and stored at −20°C this is especially advantageous in situations where adequate facilities for isolation of OAB are not readily available, as in most veterinary clinical situations.

INTRODUCTION

Reports on the bacteriology of summer mastitis are numerous and the most commonly isolated organism *Corynebacterium pyogenes* has been regarded as the main causative agent. However, this species is often not isolated in pure culture, and in recent years interest has been focused on mixed infections with non-sporulating, obligate anaerobic bacteria (OAB) (Cornelissen *et al.*, 1970; Fievez, 1965; Sorensen, 1974a; Seno and Azuma, 1983; Weber *et al.*, 1977). The pathological findings in summer mastitis, a tissue destructive inflammation with copious foul smelling pus, are also characteristic of an infection involving OAB. The classical method of evaluating the involvement of a bacterium in an infectious process is to isolate this species from pus of secretions. Another more direct way, is to demonstrate by chemical analysis of the submitted specimens the presence of structural components or characteristic metabolic endproducts. OAB characteristically produce volatile fatty acids (VFA) which are used *in vitro* for taxonomic purposes (Holdeman *et al.*, 1977). The detection of these metabolites by gas-liquid chromatography (GLC) has also been used successfully for detection of OAB in infectious processes and the presumptive diagnosis of anaerobic infections in humans (Schwan, 1975; Gorbach et al., 1976; Nord, 1977; Ladas et al., 1979) and veterinary medicine (van den Bogaard et al., 1983).

In this study, 51 secretion samples collected from affected quarters of heifers suffering from acute mastitis during the summer of 1984 and 1985 were analysed by GLC for the presence of VFA, and the data were compared with the results obtained by conventional cultural methods for isolation of OAB.

MATERIALS AND METHODS

Sampling

During the months of July and August in 1984 and 1985, twin samples of mammary secretions were collected from the affected quarters of non-lactating heifers under 2 years of age and dry cows showing clinical evidence of summer mastitis as detected by the farmer. After cleaning and disinfection of the teat, udder secretion was sampled by a veterinary surgeon via the teat canal by means of a disposable plastic syringe. After expiration of all air from the syringe and needle, a minimum of 2 ml secretion was injected into a small, gas tight, sealed bottle, containing an oxygen free atmosphere and a reducing solid medium. An equivalent volume was injected into a non-sterile, plastic tube containing approximately 1 mg of sodiumazide. Only twin samples received in the laboratory within 48 hrs of collection and containing at least 2 ml were processed. The anaerobic samples were processed immediately after arrival in an anaerobic glovebox. The samples for GLC (the plastic tubes containing sodiumazide) were stored at $-20°C$ until assayed.

Bacteriology

Smears of the secretions were stained by Gram's method. The samples were processed for isolation of (facultative) aerobic and OAB using standard procedures (Holdeman et al., 1977; van den Bogaard et al., in press).

Sample preparation for GLC-analysis

Pretreatment of summer mastitis secretions by standard methods as described previously (van den Bogaard et al., 1986) caused interfering peaks on the chromatograms and poisoning of the GLC-columns. Therefore, a special pretreatment method had to be developed. One gram of the sample was acidified with 0.1 ml of concentrated formic acid and spiked with heptanoic acid (internal standard) and thoroughly mixed with 3 ml ether. The two phases were then separated by centrifugation (2 min at 20,000 Fg) and the aqueous phase frozen (15 min at $-70°C$) before removing the ether layer: one ml 1M NaOH was added to the removed ether phase and the mixture gently shaken, subsequently centrifuged and frozen again (15 min at $-70°C$). The ether supernatant was discarded and after thawing, N_2 was flushed through the new aqueous phase to remove residual ether. It then was acidified again with concentrated formic acid to pH 2. The sample was finally centrifuged for 10 min at 20,000 Fg to remove any sediment. Samples prepared as described above, were then injected (0.2 μl) directly into the injector of the gaschromatograph.

Gas-liquid chromatography

The VFA in secretions were measured by GLC. The GLC system consisted of a Packard-Becker 433 gaschromatograph equipped with flame ionisation detectors (sensitivity 1 x 10^{-14} ampères) in conjunction with a digital processor (Packard-Becker, Delft, The Netherlands). A wide bore (25 m x 0.53 mm) WCOT fused silica column, coated with CP sil 5 CB (thickness 4.1 μm) was obtained from Chrompack B.V. (Middelburg, The Netherlands). This column was used with a temperature programme with an initial oven temperature of 55°C which was raised in 20 minutes to a final temperature of 160°C. Extra make-up gas (10 ml min^{-1} N_2) was added to the carrier gas flow (6 ml min^{-1} N_2) via a make-up Tee in front of the detector to improve sensitivity and stability. The minimum detection level of VFA (C_4-C_6) by this method was 0.02 mM and the variance in reproducibility was 4.7%. Samples were considered positive for VFA when more than 2 mM of one VFA (C_3-C_6) was detected. In milk and secretions of healthy quarters from dry heifers, more than 1 mM of any free VFA (C_3-C_6) was never detected.

RESULTS

Forty-nine of the 51 specimens examined yielded a positive culture (Table 1). In the 2 apparently sterile specimens, no bacteria could be observed by direct microscopy. In 28 specimens (55%) only (facultative) aerobes were cultured: in 12 cases (24%) in pure culture. Twenty specimens (41%) yielded a mixed culture of aerobically growing bacteria and obligate anaerobes and in one case a mixed culture of only OAB was obtained, *i.e. Peptococcus indolicus* and *Fusobacterium necrophorum*. Of the 130 isolates from 49 positive specimens, 88 (68%) were aerobic and 42 (32%) were OAB. Among the OAB, *P. indolicus* and *F. necrophorum* were most commonly isolated, in 33% and 22% respectively.

Acetic acid (C_2) was detected in nearly all specimens. All samples (n=21) which yielded OAB, were positive for VFA (C_3-C_6) except for two. From only one specimen, which was positive for propionic acid (C_3) and butyric acid (C_4), was it not possible to isolate OAB. This yielded a pure culture of *Streptococcus uberis*.

A typical example of a chromatogram of a mastitis secretion, positive for OAB on culture, is shown in Fig. 1. There was no correlation between the individual VFA detected in a OAB positive mastitis secretions and the *in vitro* production of individual VFA by the specific obligate anaerobic species isolated from these samples. Most direct Gram's stains of the secretions revealed the presence of bacteria, but their morphological features were not sufficiently clear to make a distinction between (facultative) aerobes and OAB and mixed infections were often missed.

TABLE 1. Bacteriological examination of 51 mastitis secretions obtained from heifers and dry cows during summer.

	Number	Percentage
Number of secretions examined	51	—
Sterile secretions	2	4
(Facultative) aerobic bacteria only	28	55
Obligate anaerobic bacteria only	1	2
Mixtures of aerobic and obligate anaerobic bact.	20	39
Secretions positive for volatile fatty acids (C_3-C_6)	20	39
Secretions positive for volatile fatty acids (C_4-C_6)	18	35

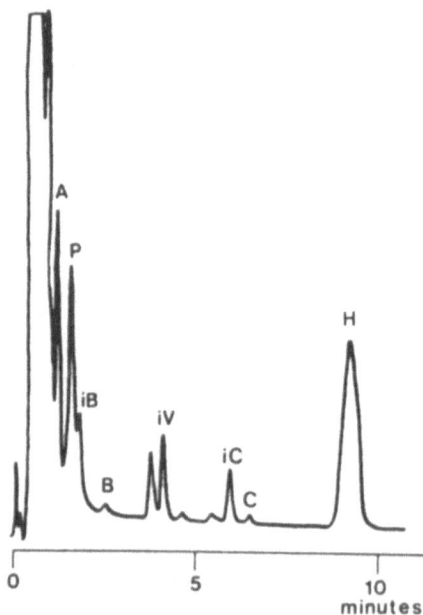

Fig. 1. Gas-chromatographic pattern of a summer mastitis secretion showing several peaks of volatile fatty acids. The peaks are: A, acetic acid (C_2); P, propionic acid (C_3); iB, iso-butyric acid (C_4); B, butyric acid (C_4); iV, iso-valeric acid (C_5); V, valeric acid (C_5); iC, iso-caproic acid (C_6); C, caproic acid (C_6); and H, heptanoic acid (C_7). Culture of this specimen yielded *Corynebacterium pyogenes*, *Peptococcus indolicus* and *Fusobacterium necrophorum*.

DISCUSSION

VFA (C_3–C_6) are metabolic products, characteristic for OAB and they can only be found in specimens taken from normally sterile tissues or sites if OAB have been metabolically active at the site of infection. Hence, OAB contaminating a specimen during sampling or processing do not give a positive VFA result. This could explain the two "false" negative cases, from which the anaerobic species could only be cultured in very low numbers or after enrichment. *Clostridium sporogenes* was isolated from one false negative, only after enrichment. This might have been an environmental contaminant. The other false negative yielded a miscellany of aerobes and anaerobes in low numbers, which strongly suggested (faecal) contamination. In this respect VFA detection by GLC might be more indicative of the involvement of OAB in an infectious process, than the isolation of one or more obligate anaerobic species from such a process. From one sample positive for VFA (C_2, C_3 and C_4), only *Streptococcus uberis* was recovered. This false positive might have been due to the fact that anaerobic species were involved which could not survive transport or could not be grown *in vitro* with the methods used.

In a previous study on swine abcesses (Van den Bogaard *et al.*, 1983) we found a better correlation between the presence of OAB and the detection of VFA (C_4–C_6). In this study however there was a better correlation with the detection of VFA (C_3–C_6). In the pus of swine abcesses, propionic acid was only detected in the absence of OAB when *E. coli* was cultured and it was presumed, that *E. coli* is capable of producing propionic acid under certain (strict anaerobic or nutritional) conditions, as might be the case in swine abcesses. Also the amounts of VFA detected in swine abcesses were higher than in the summer mastitis secretions. This might be due to dilution of the VFA produced by secretion products of the infected quarter. Propionic acid is produced by many OAB in larger amounts than other VFA (C_4–C_6). Therefore, propionic acid might in some cases have been the only VFA considered positive (> 2 mM) in some secretions, possibly because other produced VFA (C_4–C_6) were diluted below the level of 2 mM. In this study *E. coli* was only isolated from one secretion, which also yielded *Staph. epidermis*, but no OAB and which was also negative for VFA.

CONCLUSION

This study shows a good correlation between the detection of VFA (C_3–C_6) by GLC and culture of OAB. This suggests not only that detection of VFA (C_3–C_6) by GLC is highly indicative for the presence of OAB in these samples, but also the involvement of these OAB in the infectious process.

SUMMER MASTITIS: BACTERIOLOGICAL ASPECTS

J. Reichmuth and G. Hahn

Institut für Hygiene,
Bundesanstalt für Milchforschung,
D 2300 Kiel, F.R.G.

ABSTRACT

The bacteriological results from 88 typical cases of summer mastitis in heifers (Schleswig-Holstein, summer 1981 and 1982) are reported: *C. pyogenes* = 77 (87,5%); *C. pyogenes* + *P. indolicus* +/or Bacteroidaceae = 69 (78,4%); no isolation of anaerobes = 15 (17%). The bacteriological results from suppurative wounds in 5 grazing cows in an area without summer mastitis reported during the same summer (1982) showed the same species as isolated from summer mastitis but in different combinations.

INTRODUCTION

Research on the bacteriological implications of summer mastitis led to two aspects amongst others:

— From the pathognomonic udder secretion several species of microorganisms (aerobes and anaerobes) can be isolated in a variety of different combinations;

— the same variety of species and combinations seem to colonize bovines in different parts of the body normally and/or also play a role in other pathological processes.

The following data add to these findings. They are part of a study published elsewhere (Tolle *et al.*, 1985).

BACTERIOLOGICAL RESULTS FROM FIELD CASES OF SUMMER MASTITIS

The bacteriological results from 88 typical cases of summer mastitis in heifers (Schleswig-Holstein, summer 1981 and 1982) are given in Table 1 with regard to species and combinations.

The percentage of *C. pyogenes* (87,5%) in combination with *P. indolicus* and/or Bacteroidaceae (78,4%) is high; only 15 cases (17%) were without isolations of anaerobes.

BACTERIOLOGICAL RESULTS FROM WOUNDS IN GRAZING GOWS

Extirpations of fat (dorsally near the shoulder-blade) were carried out in grazing cows for residue assay.

In 5 of the cows suppurative processes developed. The bacteriological results from these wounds (swabs) are given in Table 2.

TABLE 1.   Bacteria isolated from summer mastitis (88 cases)

Bacteria	n	Cases percentage	Bacteria	n	Cases percentage
C + P + Scd	11		P + Scd	3	4,6%
C + P	16	65,9%	P + B + Scd	1	
C + P + B	18		others	7	7.9%
C + P + B + Scd	13	78,4%			
C + B	8	47,7%			
C + B + Scd	3				
C + others	4				
C + Scd	2	9,1%			
C	2				
Total	**77**	**87,5%**		**11**	**12.5%**

Micrococcus spp: 27 cases (31%) in different combinations

C = *C. pyogenes*	Scd = *Sc. dysgalactiae*
P = *P. indolicus*	B = *Bacteroidaceae*

TABLE 2.   Bacteria from suppurative wounds in grazing cows

Cow	C	P	B	Scd	M	others
1191	+	+		+		+
1196	+			+	+	
1135	+		+	+		
1032	+	+			+	+
631	+				+	+

C = *C. pyogenes*	Scd = *Sc. dysgalactiae*
P = *P. indolicus*	B = Bacteroidaceae
	M = *Micrococcus* spp.

These findings add to those which indicate the general presence of all the microorganisms involved in summer mastitis in and/or around the bovine. No case of summer mastitis was reported during the summer (1982) in the area of the experimental farm where the cows were kept.

70

REFERENCES

Aalbaek, B. 1971. *Sphaerophorus necrophorus*. A study of 23 strains. Act. Vet. Scand., **12**, 344-364.

Aalbaek, B. 1973. Bacteroidaceae. Status of classification and identification of anaerobic, non-sporing gram-negative rods. Nord. Vet.-Med., **25**, 409-419.

Aalbaek, B. 1978. On the occurrence of *Fusobacterium necrophorum* in bovine mastitis. Nord. Vet.-Med., **30**, 231-232.

Anon. 1982. Kommission zur Erarbeitung von Richtlinien für die mikrobiologische Diagnostik. Isolierung und Identifizierung von *Corynebacterium, Listeria* und *Erysipelothrix*. Zbl. Bakt. Hyg. I. Abt. Orig. A, **253**, 43-60.

Bahr, L. 1952. Nogle undersogelser vedrorende "sommermastitis". Forste beretning. (Some investigations on "summer mastitis". First report.) Dansk Månedsskr. Dyrl., **62**, 367-394.

Berg, J.N. and Loan, R.W. 1975. *Fusobacterium necrophorum* and *Bacteroides melaninogenicus* as etiologic agents of foot rot in cattle. Am. J. Vet. Res., **36**, 1115-1122.

Biberstein, E.L., Knight, H.D. and England, K. 1968. *Bacteroides melaninogenicus* in diseases of domestic animals. J. A. V. M. A., **153**, 1045-1049.

Bock, R. 1980. Nachweis von *C. pyogenes* in Tonsillen und Lymphknoten von gesunden Kälbern und Jungrindern und dessen Bedeutung für das Auftreten der Sommermastitis. Diss., Hannover.

Bogaard, A.E.J.M. van den, Hazen, M.J. and Maes, J.H.J. 1983. The detection of obligate anaerobic bacteria in swine abcesses. A comparison between gas-liquid chromatography and bacteriological culturing methods. Vet. Microbiol., **8**, 389-396.

Bogaard, A.E.J.M. van den, Hazen, M.J. and van Boven, C.P. 1986. Quantitative gas chromatographic analysis of volatile fatty acids in spent culture media and body fluids. J. Clin. Microbiol., **23**, 523-530.

Bogaard, A.E.J.M. van den, Hazen, H.J. and Vecht, U. 1986. The detection of obligate anaerobic bacteria in udder secretions of heifers and dry cows during summer. Vet. Microbiol., in press.

Bourgault, A.M. and Rosenblatt, J.E. 1979. First isolation of *Peptococcus indolicus* from a human clinical specimen. J. Clin. Microbiol., **9**, 549-550.

Bramley, A.J., Leaver, J.D., Kingwill, R.G. and Simpkin, D.L. 1977. *Corynebacterium pyogenes* mastitis among heifer calves. Vet. Rec., **100**, 464-465.

Bramley, A.J., Hillerton, J.E., Higgs, T.M. and Hogben, E.M. 1985. The carriage of summer mastitis pathogens by muscid flies. Br. Vet. J., **141**, 618-627.

Brook, I., Hunter, V. and Walker, R.I. 1984. Synergistic effect of *Bacteroides, Clostridium, Fusobacterium*, anaerobic cocci, and aerobic bacteria on mortality and induction of subcutaneous abscesses in mice. J. Infect. Dis., **149**, 924-929.

Cameron, C.M. and Fuls, W.J.P. 1977. Failure to induce in rabbits effective immunity to a mixed infection of *Fusobacterium necrophorum* and *Corynebacterium pyogenes* with a combined bacterin. Onderstepoort. J. Vet. Res., **44**, 253-256.

Carlsson, J., Höfling, J.F. and Sundqvist, G.K. 1984. Degradation of albumin, haemopexin, haptoglobin and transferrin, by black-pigmented *Bacteroides* species. J. Med. Microbiol., **18**, 39-46.

Chirino-Trejo, J.M. and Prescott, J.F. 1983. The identification and antimicrobial susceptibility of anaerob bacteria from pneumonic cattle lungs. Can. J. Comp. Med., **47**, 270-276.

Christiansen, M. 1934. Ein obligat anaerober, gasbildender, Indol positiver Micrococcus. Act. Path. Microbiol. Scand. Suppl., **18**, 42-63.

Cornelisse, J.L., Saes, J.M.F. and Attenveld, J.C. 1970. De isolatie van anaerobe pepto-streptokokken, uit uiersecretum van runderen met wrang. Tijdschr. Diergeneesk., **95**, 387-391.

Cowan, S.T. and Steel, K.J. 1974. Manual for the identification of medical bacteria. Cambridge University Press, Cambridge, 238 pp.

Daniel, R.C.W., Barnum, D.A. and Leslie, K.E. 1986. Observations on intramammary infections in first calf heifers in early lactation. Can. Vet. J., **27**, 112-115.

Du Preez, J.H., Greeff, A.S. and Eksteen, N. 1981. Isolation and significance of anaerobic bacteria isolated from cases of bovine mastitis. Onderstepoort J. Vet. Res., **48**, 123-126.

Du Preez, J.H., Greeff, A.S. and Botha, W.S. 1982. Pathology of the bovine udder parenchyma caused by asporogenous obligate anaerobic bacteria isolated from cases of bovine mastitis. J. of the S.A. Vet. Ass., **3**, 157-159.

Emery, D.L., Dufty, J.H. and Clark, B.L. 1984. Biochemical and functional properties of a leucocidin produced by several strains of *Fusobacterium necrophorum*. Aust. Vet. J., **61**, 382-387.

Everz, K.-E. and Linge, F. 1975. Kvigmastiter på Gotland. En preliminär undersöknings-rapport. Svensk Veterinärtidning, **27**, 660-662.

Ezaki, T., Yamamoto, N., Ninomiya, K., Suzuki, S. and Yabuuchi, E. 1983. Transfer of *Peptococcus indolicus, Peptococcus asaccharolyticus, Peptococcus prevotii*, and *Peptococcus magnus* to the genus *Peptostreptococcus* and proposal of *Peptostreptococcus tetradius* sp. nov. Int. J. Syst. Bacteriol., **33**, 683-698.

Fiévez, L. 1963. Etude comparée des souches de *Sphaerophorus necrophorus* isolées chez l'Homme et chez l'Animal. Presses Acad. Europ., Bruxelles.

Fiévez, L. 1965. Association de bacteries pyogenes anaerobies non sporulées et de *Corynebacterium pyogenes* dans les pus des absces mammaires de la vache. Ann. Med. Vet., **109**, 389-408.

Francis, J. 1941. A bacteriological examination of bovine tonsils and vaginas. The possible relationship of the findings to mastitis and pneumonia. Br. Vet. J., **97**, 243-251.

Franke, V., Tolle, A., Reichmuth, J. and Beimgraben, J. 1983. Heifer mastitis in Schleswig-Holstein/FRG — situation, bacteriology, prevention. Heifer Mastitis Seminar, Stockholm-Helsinki.

Fujimura, S. and Nakamura, T. 1981. Isolation and characterization of proteases from *Bacteroides melaninogenicus*. Infect. Immun., **23**, 738-742.

Glage, F. 1903. Über den *Bacillus pyogenes suis* Grips, den *Bacillus pyogenes bovis* Künne-mann und den bakteriologischen Befund bei den chronischen, abscedierenden Euterentzündungen der Milchkühe. Zschr. Fleisch. Milchhyg., **13**, 166-175.

Glage, F. 1908. Holsteinische Euterseuche. Berl. Tierärztl. Wschr., **48**, 862-863.

Gorbach, S.L., Mayhew, J.W., Batlett, J.G. and Onderdonk, A.B. 1976. Rapid diagnosis of anaerobic infections by gas-liquid chromatography. J. Clin. Invest., **57**, 478-484.

Greeff, A.S., Du Preez, J.H. and de Beer, Maria. 1983. The frequency and some characteristics of anaerobic bacteria isolated from various forms of bovine mastitis. J. S.A. Vet. Ass., **1**, 25-28.

Grupe, W. 1963. Untersuchungen von Rindertonsillen auf das Vorkommen von *Corynebacterium pyogenes*. Diss., Berlin.

Hansen, J. and Nielsen, S.A. 1983. Summermastitis. A review. Heifer Mastitis Seminar, Stockholm-Helsinki.

Hartwigk, H. 1980. *Corynebacterium pyogenes*. In "Handbuch der bakteriellen Infektionen bei Tieren" (Eds. H. Blobel und T. Schliesser). (Gustav Fischer Verlag, Stuttgart). pp. 279-323.

Heinrich, S., Pulverer, G. and Hanf, U. 1959. Uber das physiologische Vorkommen des *Bacteroides melaninogenicus* bei Mensch und Tier. Schweiz. Z. Path. Bakt., **22**, 861-870.

Hillerton, J.E., Bramley, A.J. and Broom, D.M. 1983. *Hydrotaea irritans* and summer mastitis in calves. Vet. Rec., **113**, 88.

Holdeman, L.V., Cato, E.P. and Moore, W.E.C. 1977. Anaerobe Laboratory Manual 4th ed. Virginia Polytechnic Institute and State University, Blacksburg, Virginia.

Horsch, F., Nattermann, H., Dietz, O. and Koch, K. 1974. Die *Corynebacterium pyogenes* Infektion des Rindes. I. Mitt. Bakteriologie und Pathogenese. Mh. Vet.-Med., **29**, 807-813.

Ingham, H.R., Selkon, J.B., So, S.C. and Weiser, R. 1975. Brain abscess. Brit. Med. J., **4**, 39-40.

Jorgensen, K. Leth. 1937. Mastitis fremkaldt af Blandingsinfektion med *Bacterium pyogenes* og anaerobe Mikrokokker. (Mastitis caused by a mixed infection with *Bacterium pyogenes* and anaerobic micrococci). Maanedsskr. Dyrl., **49**, 113-129.

Karmann, P. 1928. Die Weideeuterentzündung der Kühe und Färsen in Ostfriesland. Z. Inf. Krkh. Haust., **34**, 122-152.

Kasper, D.L. and Finegold, S.M. 1979. Virulence factors of anaerobic bacteria. Rev. Infect. Dis., **1**, 245-400.

Kaufman, E.J., Mashimo, P.A., Hausmann, E., Hanks, C.T. and Ellison, S.A. 1972. Fusobacterial infection: Enhancement by cell free extracts of *Bacteroides melaninogenicus* possessing collagenolytic activity. Archs. Oral Biol., **17**, 577-580.

Klastrup, O. and Schmidt-Madsen, P. 1974. Nordiske rekommendationer vedrorende mastitundersogelser af kirtelprover. Nord. Vet.-Med., **26**, 197-204.

Ladas, S., Arapakis, G., Mamalou, H., Palikaris, G. and Arseni, A. 1979. Rapid diagnosis of anaerobic infections by gas-liquid chromatography. J. Clin. Pathol., **32**, 1163-1167.

LaLiberté, M. and Mayrand, D. 1983. Characterization of black-pigmented *Bacteroides* strains isolated from animals. J. Appl. Bacteriol., **55**, 247-252.

Langhorn, E. 1910. Om Mastitis hos Efteraarskaelvere i Goldperioden. (On mastitis in autumn calvers in the dry period). Maanedsskr. Dyrl. **XXII**, 240-242.

Langworth, B.F. 1977. *Fusobacterium necrophorum*: Its characteristics and role as an animal pathogen. Bacteriol. Rev., **41**, 373-390.

Lee, S.W., Alexander, B. and McGowan, B. 1983. Purification, characterization, and serologic characteristics of *Bacteroides nodosus* pili and use of a purified pili vaccine in sheep. Amer. J. Vet. Res., **44**, 1676-1681.

Lipton, M.E. and Isalska, B.J. 1983. *Corynebacterium pyogenes meningitis*. J. Neurology, Neurosurgery & Psychiatry, **46**, 873-874.

Lovell, R. 1937. Studies on *Corynebacterium pyogenes* with special reference to toxin production. J. Path. Bact., **45**, 339-355.

Madsen, M. 1985. Sommermastitis. Bakteriologiske og transmissionsdynamiske undersogelser. (Investigations on the bacteriology and transmission dynamics of summer mastitis in cattle). Ph. D. thesis, Copenhagen.

Madsen, M., Sorensen, G. Hoi and Aalbaek, B. 1985. Bakteriologiske undersogelser af sekreter fra akutte tilfaelde af sommermastitis. (Bacteriological examinations of secretions from acute cases of summer mastitis). In "Initiativet: Sommermastitis" (Ed. P. Nansen) (Report to the Danish Agricultural and Veterinary Research Council, Copenhagen)., pp. 20-27.

Marshall, A.B. 1981. Summer mastitis. NIRD Techn. Bull., **4**, 81-94.

McGillivery, D.J. and Nicholls, T.J. 1984. Isolation of *Fusobacterium necrophorum* from a case of bovine mastitis. Aust. Vet. J., **61**, 325.

Michael, L. 1983. Untersuchungen symboviner Fliegen auf *Corynebacterium pyogenes* unter besonderer Berücksichtigung der Sommermastitis. Diss., Hannover.

Müller, H.E. 1973. Neuraminidase und acylneuraminat-pyruvatlyase bei *Corynebacterium haemolyticum* und *Corynebacterium pyogenes*. Zbl. Bakt. Hyg. I. Abt. Orig. A, **225**, 59-65.

Nansen, P. (Ed.) 1985. Initiativet: Sommermastitis. (The initiative: Summer mastitis.) Report to the Danish Agricultural and Veterinary Research Council, Cogenhagen.

Nattermann, H. and Horsch, F. 1977. Die *Corynebacterium pyogenes*-Infektion des Rindes. I. Mitteilung: Verbreitung des Erregers. Arch. Exp. Vet.-Med., **31**, 405-413.

Nord, C.E. 1979. Diagnosis of anaerobic infections by gas-liquid chromatography. Acta Pathol. Microbiol. Scand., sect. B, **259**, 55-59.

Norenberg, D.D., Bigley, V., Virata, R.L. and Liang, G.C. 1978. *Corynebacterium pyogenes* septic arthritis with plasma cell synovial infiltrate and monoclonal gammopathy. Arch. Int. Med., **138**, 810-811.

Ohm, B. 1958. Infektion des infantilen Rindereuters. Diss., Giessen.

Olsson, S.-O., Jonsson, P., Holmberg, O. and Funke, H. 1986. Heifer mastitis in Sweden during a three year period (1982-1985). Background and some preliminary data on the incidence of heifer mastitis. Proc. from "EEC workshop on summer mastitis", 23-24 Oct., 1986, Lelystad, Nl.

Poels, J. 1910. De uierziekten van het rund, het schaap en de geit. Tijdschr. Veeartsenijk., **37**, 789-824.

Roberts, D.S. 1967a. The pathogenic synergy of *Fusiformis necrophorus* and *Corynebacterium pyogenes*. I. Influence of the leucocidal exotoxin of *F. necrophorus*. Brit. J. Exp. Path., **48**, 665-673.

Roberts, D.S. 1967b. The pathogenic synergy of *Fusiformis necrophorus* and *Corynebacterium pyogenes*. II. The response of *F. necrophorus* to a filterable product of *C. pyogenes*, Brit. J. Exp. Path., **48**, 674-679.

Roberts, D.S., Graham, N.P.H. and Egerton, J.R. 1968. Infective bulbar necrosis (heel-abscess) of sheep, a mixed infection with *Fusiformis necrophorus* and *Corynebacterium pyogenes*. J. Comp. Path., **78**, 1-8.

Saes, J.M.F. 1970. Voorkomen, pathogenese en bestrijding van *Corynebacterium pyogenes* mastitis (wrang) bij runderen in Limburg. Diss., Utrecht.

Saes, J.M.F. 1971. Voorkomen, pathogenese en bestrijding van *C. pyogenes*-mastitis (wrang) bij runderen in Limbrug. Tijdschr. Diergeneesk., **96**, 1306-1317.

Schmidt, H.M. 1910. Yverbetaendelse i Eftersommeren. (Mastitis in late summer). Maanedsskr. Dyrl. **XXII**, 466-470.

Schmidt Madsen, P., Klastrup, O., Olsen, Sv.J. and Stovlbaek Pederson, P. 1974. Herd incidence of bovine mastitis in four Danish dairy districts. I. The prevalence and mastitogenic effect of microorganisms in the mammary glands of cows. Nord. Vet.-Med., **26**, 473-482.

Schwan, O. 1975. Preliminär undersökung rörande förekomst av anaerobe bakterier i mastimjölk hos nötkreatur. Svensk Veterinärtidning, **27**, 654-659.

Schwan, O. 1979a. Heifer mastitis and dry cow mastitis. Bacteriological and serological investigations with special reference to mixed infection with *Corynebacterium pyogenes, Peptococcus indolicus* and microaerophilic cocci. Thesis, Uppsala.

Schwan, O. 1979b. Biochemical, enzymatic, and serological differentiation of *Peptococcus indolicus* (Christiansen) Sorensen from *Peptococcus asaccharolyticus* (Distaso) Douglas. J. Clin. Microbiol., **9**, 157-162.

Schwan, O. 1980. IgG antibody response to *Corynebacterium pyogenes, Peptococcus indolicus* and microaerophilic cocci in natural and experimental mastitis. Vet. Microbiol., **5**, 19-34.

Schwan, O. and Holmberg, O. 1978/1979. Heifer mastitis and dry cow mastitis. A bacteriological survey in Sweden. Vet. Microbiol., **3**, 213-226.

Schwan, O. and Smyth, C.J. 1980. Crossed immunoelectrophoretic analysis of the antibody response in heifers and dry cows to *Peptococcus indolicus* in experimental and natural heifer mastitis and dry cow mastitis. Vet. Microbiol., **5**, 57-72.

Schwan, O., Nord, C.E. and Holmberg, O. 1979. Biochemical characterization of unidentified microaerophilic cocci isolated from heifer mastitis and dry cow mastitis. J. Clin. Microbiol., **10**, 622-627.

Seno, N. and Azuma, R. 1983. A study on heifer mastitis in Japan and its causative microorganisms. Natl. Inst. Anim. Health (Jpn), **32**, 82-91.

Shimizu, T., Shinjo, T., Hamana, K., Nagamoto, H., Nosaka, D., Otsuka, H., Hataya, M., Sakanoshita, A. and Shindo, H. 1975. Studies on the heifer mastitis. Biochemical properties and microbiological findings of exudates from normal and mastitic udders of the heifer. Bull. Facult. Agricult. Miyazaki Univ., **22**, 131-139.

Shinjo, T. 1983. *Fusobacterium necrophorum* isolated from a hepatic abscess and from udder secretions in a heifer. Ann. Microbiol. Inst. Pasteur, **134 B**, 401-409.

Shinjo, T., Shimizu, T., Nagamoto, H., Nosaka, D., Hamana, K., Otsuka, H., Hataya, M., Sakanoshita, A. and Shindo, H. 1976. Studies on the heifer mastitis. III. Bacteriological examination of mastitic and normal udders of affected heifers. Bull. Facult. Agricult. Miyazaki Univ., **23**, 219-223.

Simon, P.C. and Stovell, P.L. 1969. Diseases of animals associated with *Sphaerophorus necrophorus*: Characteristics of the organism. Vet. Bull., **39**, 311-315.

Slee, K.J. 1985. A microaerophilic coccus in pyogenic infections of ruminants. Aust. Vet. J., **62**, 57-59.

Slee, K.J. and McOrist, S. 1985. Mastitis due to a group of pyogenic bacteria. Aust. Vet. J., **62**, 63-65.

Skovgaard, N. 1968. The incidence of hemolytic bacteria in cattle with a special view to *Corynebacterium pyogenes* as the causative agent of "Summer Mastitis". Yearbook, Royal Veterinary and Agricultural University, Copenhagen., pp. 89-108.

Smyth, C.J., Zimmermann, E.K. and Schwan, O. 1980. Antigenic analysis of *Peptococcus indolicus* by crossed immunoelectrophoresis. Vet. Microbiol., **5**, 35-56.

Sol, J., Vecht, U., Thomas, G. 1985. Summer mastitis: incidence bacteriology, aetiology. Methods of Prevention and entomological aspects. Kiel. Milch. Forschung., **37**, 593-600.

Sorensen, G. Hoi. 1972a. Sommermastitis — eksperimentelt fremkaldt hos juvenile kvier. (Summer mastitis — experimentally reproduced in juvenile heifers). Nord. Vet.-Med., **24**, 247-258.

Sorensen, G. Hoi. 1972b. Sommermastitis. Den mulige beskyttende virkning af to forskellige vacciner over for eksperimentelle infektioner. (Summer mastitis. The possible protective effect of two different vaccines against experimental infection.) Nord. Vet.-Med., 24, 259-271.

Sorensen, G. Hoi. 1973. *Micrococcus indolicus*. Some biochemical properties, and the demonstration of six antigenically different types. Act. Vet. Scand., 14, 301-326.

Sorensen, G. Hoi. 1974a. Studies on the aetiology and transmission of summer mastitis. Nord. Vet.-Med., 26, 122-133.

Sorensen, G. Hoi. 1974b. *Corynebacterium pyogenes*. A biochemical and serological study. Act. Vet. Scand., 15, 544-554.

Sorensen, G. Hoi. 1974c. *Peptococcus indolicus*. Its occurrence, identification and classification. XI Conf. Taxonomy Bacteria, Brno, 1974.

Sorensen, G. Hoi. 1975. *Peptococcus* (s. *Micrococcus*) *indolicus*. The demonstration of two varieties of hemolysin forming strains. Act. Vet. Scand., 16, 218-225.

Sorensen, G. Hoi. 1976. Studies on the occurrence of *Peptococcus indolicus* and *Corynebacterium pyogenes* in apparently healthy cattle. Act. Vet. Scand., 17, 15-24.

Sorensen, G. Hoi. 1978a. Bacteriological examination of summer mastitis secretions. The demonstration of Bacteroidaceae. Nord. Vet.-Med., 30, 199-204.

Sorensen, G. Hoi. 1978b. Studies on the occurrence of *Peptococcus indolicus* and *Corynebacterium pyogenes* in swine abscesses and on the occurrence of *Peptococcus indolicus* in apparently normal skin and mucous membranes of piglets. Nord. Vet.-Med., 30, 282-285.

Sorensen, G. Hoi. 1979. Sommermastitis. (Summer mastitis.) Thesis, Copenhagen.

Sorensen, G. Hoi. 1980. Comparative studies on *Corynebacterium pyogenes* toxin formation in monocultures and mixed cultures — the demonstration of a stimulating effect of *Peptococcus indolicus* and Stuart-Schwan cocci. Act. Vet. Scand., 21, 438-448.

Stuart, P., Buntain, D. and Langridge, R.G. 1951. Bacteriological examination of secretions from cases of "Summer Mastitis" and experimental infections of non-lactating bovine udders. Vet. Rec., 63, 451-453.

Switalski, L.M., Schwan, O., Smyth, C.J. and Wadström, T. 1978. Peptocoagulase: Clotting factor produced by bovine strains of *Peptococcus indolicus*. J. Clin. Microbiol., 7, 361-367.

Takeuchi, S., Azuma, R. and Suto, T. 1979. Purification and some properties of hemolysin produced by *Corynebacterium pyogenes*. Jap. J. Vet. Sci., 41, 511-516.

Tolle, A., Franke, V. and Reichmuth, J. 1983. Zur *C. pyogenes*-Mastitis — Bakteriologische Aspekte. Dtsch. Tierärztl. Wschr., 90, 256-260.

Tolle, A., Reichmuth, J., Franke, V. and Beimgraben, J. 1985. Untersuchungen zur Pyogenes-Mastitis des Rindes (Studies on bovine summer mastitis). Kiel. Milch. Forschung., 36 (2), 125-212.

Weber, A., Schliesser, T. and Steiner, G. 1977. Zum kulturellen Nachweis von anaeroben Kokken, insbesondere vom *Micrococcus indolicus* in Milchsekretproben von Rindern mit Pyogenes-Mastitis. Dtsch. Tierärztl. Wschr., 84, 165-167.

Yanagawa, R. and Honda, E. 1976. Presence of pili in species of human and animal parasites and pathogens of the genus *Corynebacterium*. Infect. Immun., 13, 1293-1295.

DISCUSSION

From the discussion following the session of bacteriology it appeared that a proper definition of summer mastitis is still lacking. Depending on the discipline concerned, different definitions were proposed: the epidemiologist, the bacteriologist and the entomologist tend to diagnose with different criteria. It was generally accepted that a definition of summer mastitis should be based on both bacteriological and epidemiological criteria.

The criteria for bacteriological diagnosis are still unclear as a variety of bacteria are isolated from field cases. *Corynebacterium pyogenes* and obligate anaerobic bacteria (OAB) such as *Peptococcus indolicus, Fusobacterium necrophorum*, and *Bacteroides* species are often isolated, although in varying frequencies in the last years in different countries. *Streptococcus dysgalactiae* is also an example of this and was, in the past, more often isolated in the United Kingdom than at present, probably due to changes in therapy policies or housing conditions. Even the involvement of *C. pyogenes* was questioned, due to varying isolation rates and the identical response to therapy in cases where OAB were isolated, with or without *C. pyogenes*. It was argued that for diagnosis of summer mastitis, serology alone, *e.g.* to demonstrate the presence of antihemolysins, is not sufficient.

The variation in bacteriological results could also be due to the fact that little is known of the sequence of infection *in vivo*. It was speculated that *C. pyogenes* might act as a precursor, promoting growth of other bacteria such as OAB, which would in turn account for the more severe lesions encountered in a classical case of summer mastitis.

Interaction between the various bacteria is also considered to play a role in the pathogenesis of the disease. This would partly explain the differences in number of bacteria required to establish infection under experimental conditions as compared to the situation in the field. Another explanation might be the differences within bacterial species in virulence factors such as the presence of pili, production of various enzymes and toxins. It was felt that in order to develop a satisfactory scheme for therapy and control of summer mastitis these bacteriological aspects deserve research.

Response to therapy is poor, especially when OAB are involved. Moreover, the bacteria are not easily eliminated from the mammary gland tissue. To explain the endemic character of summer mastitis in herds the observation was reported that 2 to 3 years after clinical disease *C. pyogenes* could still be isolated from mammary secretions. This suggests a very long period of excretion, in which an animal could be a source of contamination for others.

Some minor issues, which were discussed are:

(a) Definition of microaerophilic cocci; gram positive, katalase negative cocci, which are more easily isolated from primary culture when grown under anaerobic conditions, but resistant against metronidazole.

(b) Transportation of samples for anaerobe bacteriology; possible with commercially available transport media, but also the sample itself, being the typical summer mastitis excretion, is very suitable provided that no air is trapped within the vial/tube. Optimal temperature for transportation is 15°C. Processing in the laboratory should start within 24 hours of sampling.

3. AETIOLOGY AND PATHOGENESIS

Chairmen A.J. Bramley & U. Vecht

AETIOLOGY AND PATHOGENESIS OF SUMMER MASTITIS

A.J. Bramley

Milking and Mastitis Centre,
AFRC Institute for Research on Animal Disease,
Compton, Berks, RG16 0NN, U.K.

ABSTRACT

The complex microbial aetiology of summer mastitis is described with respect to field cases and the evidence of pathogenicity of the various organisms from experimental infections. Data implicating cattle flies in transmission are reviewed and the factors possibly influencing the establishment of intramammary infection discussed. Finally clinical and laboratory diagnosis are reviewed and possible approaches to rapid diagnosis suggested.

AETIOLOGY

Summer mastitis has probably affected dairy cows of northern Europe for centuries. Clear descriptions of the disease are found in the literature of the early 20th. century and colloquial names abound (Bean *et al.*, 1943). The aetiology of the disease has only been established more recently and has been discovered to be more complex as more subtle methods of microbiological analysis have been applied. Up to the 1950s the causative organism was believed to be *Actinomyces pyogenes*, formerly known as *Corynebacterium pyogenes*, although *Streptococcus dysgalactiae* was also frequently isolated from the secretions (Munch-Peterson, 1938). However Jorgensen (1937) reported the isolation of anaerobic cocci from cases and suggested a symbiosis with *A. pyogenes*. Stuart, Buntain and Langridge (1951) produce further evidence of the involvement of an anaerobic coccus and also isolated a microaerophilic coccus in addition to *A. pyogenes* and *Str. dysgalactiae*. The anaerobic coccus was identified as *Peptococcus indolicus*, now termed *Peptostreptococcus indolicus*, but the taxonomic position of the microaerophile is uncertain. The studies of Schwan *et al.* (1979) and our own unpublished observations indicate a relatively high homogeneity among the isolates however.

Several other studies broadly confirmed the findings of Stuart *et al.* (1951) but Sorensen (1978) demonstrated that other anaerobes may also be present, notably *Bacteroides melanogenicus* and *Fusobacterium necrophorum*. This has subsequently been confirmed in other studies, particularly where strict methods of anaerobic sample collection and examination have been employed (Du Preez *et al.*, 1981). It remains possible that future studies will reveal an even more complex flora, possibly involving mycoplasmas or viruses (Gibbs, 1986).

Thus we are presented with a range of bacteria which may be present in field cases. Determination of the pathogenicity of these bacteria requires their use, individually or in combination, to reproduce the clinical disease. Several studies have addressed this problem but success has usually been judged in clinical not in pathological terms. Stuart *et al.* (1951) challenged mammary glands with various combinations of *A. pyogenes, P. indolicus, Str. dysgalactiae* and the microaerophilic coccus. They broadly concluded that all these bacteria contributed to pathogenicity and that monocultures of *A. pyogenes* generally failed to reproduce the clinical disease. Sorensen (1974) infected heifers and his results indicated that the "minimum requirement" was *A. pyogenes* and *P. indolicus* although again other organisms appeared to contribute. The interpretation of these studies is difficult. *A. pyogenes* is, *per se*, pathogenic but the severity of the disease produced is lower than field cases. *Str. dysgalactiae* is a well established mastitis pathogen and even *P. indolicus* can produce clinical disease, (Hillerton, 1985).

It may be reasonable to consider the haemolytic and toxic activity of *A. pyogenes* as the prime factor in the pathological changes during summer mastitis. If so, the presence of other organisms may contribute to virulence by stimulating growth or toxin elaboration by *A. pyogenes* or by providing additional toxins or enzymes contributing to tissue damage. Using peritoneal inoculation of the mouse Tolle & Reichmuth (1985) reported that *A. pyogenes* alone, or combined with *P. indolicus*, gave similar lethality. The inclusion of *F. necrophorum* increased deaths considerably. *P. indolicus* and the microaerophilic coccus appear to increase toxin production by *C. pyogenes in vitro* (Sorensen, 1980) and this may be significant although further work is needed both *in vitro* and *in vivo*. Such studies will be aided by rapid and accurate methods to quantify *C. pyogenes* toxin and other toxins, haemolysins etc. produced by the other organisms.

PATHOGENESIS

Under this heading two aspects will be considered. Firstly, evidence for the involvement of an insect vector in transmission and secondly, the sequence of events which may occur in the infection process.

Transmission of infection

Anecdotal and circumstantial evidence of cattle flies in summer mastitis transmission is strong but nevertheless should be kept in perspective. Cases of summer mastitis occur throughout the year and thus in circumstances, when flies cannot be involved. For most of the year such cases are sporadic and it is between July and September in Northern Europe that outbreaks of the disease occur. This suggests either a vast increase in the population at risk over the critical period or the existence of a transmission or exposure mechanism occurring uniquely at that time. With autumn-calving herds there is an increase in the numbers of non-lactating cattle over this period. This is less marked for heifers and calves or where spring calving predominates (*e.g.* Ireland).

In addition there is evidence of a transmission mechanism operating over the summer. The incidence of summer mastitis varies topographically and these variations correlate with densities of fly populations (Hansen and Nielsen, 1983). Fly populations peak over the critical period of July to September, and *Hydrotaea irritans*, the predominant fly species visiting the teats and udder, occurs in the countries suffering the epidemic form of the disease (Hillerton *et al.*, 1984). Furthermore, *H. irritans* carry the relevant bacteria, (Bramley *et al.*, 1985) are attracted to mastitic animals to feed on the teats and acquire pathogenic organisms in the process (Hillerton *et al.*, 1983). *H. irritans* will migrate over several kilometers, permitting spread between herds (Robinson and Luff, 1979) and can retain the bacteria in the gut for several days (Wright and Titchener, 1977). It has also been found that infected flies can contaminate a surface by regurgitation of gut contents during feeding although there are doubts about whether the dose of organisms delivered in this way is adequate for infection (Hillerton, unpublished data).

Summer mastitis occurs more frequently in front quarters (Hillerton *et al.*, 1986a) possibly because these quarters are more accessible to the fly and less protected by fly-dislodging flicks of the tail (Hillerton *et al.*, 1986b). Control of flies by insecticides, by retaining cattle indoors or by teat bandaging to prevent fly contact appear to reduce summer mastitis incidence (Tolle and Reichmuth, 1985). A crucial stage in the hypothesis is the unequivocal demonstration that *H. irritans* can transmit the disease from infected to uninfected cattle. Tarry, Wilson and Stuart (1978) reported such an experiment but our group and others in Europe have been unable to reproduce this in recent trials.

Pathogenesis of intramammary infection

Detailed information on the stages in the establishment of a summer mastitis infection are lacking. For most udder disease the initial stage in infection is the entry of bacteria into the mammary gland via the teat duct. It is tempting to assume that such a mechanism also operates for summer mastitis. There are however significant differences between summer mastitis and most other forms of intramammary infection. Firstly it has a complex aetiology and, secondly, it frequently affects heifers and young stock prior to first calving. At this stage a particularly effective teat barrier to infection might be anticipated. It seems improbable that infection with the various pathogens involved in the disease occurs simultaneously. A succession of events seems more likely. At Compton we have been able to superimpose *A. pyogenes* in quarters infected with *P. indolicus* and vice versa. Egan (1985) suggested that the initial event in summer mastitis was infection with *Str. dysgalactiae* or one of the other common mastitis pathogens. Possibly these initial invaders are then subsequently eliminated but many summer mastitis infections are found in which *Str. dysgalactiae, Staphylococcus aureus* etc. are not detected (Sorensen, 1974; Hillerton *et al.*, 1986b). In our experiments contamination of the teat surface with *A. pyogenes* or

Str. dysgalactiae will lead to intramammary infection. Similar exposure to *P. indolicus* has not. This may suggest that *P. indolicus* enters not via the teat duct but by some other route. *P. indolicus* can be isolated from mucous membranes, tonsils and other lymphoid tissue and from a range of abscesses in cattle and pigs (Sorensen, 1976a). Intramammary infection with *A. pyogenes* can also be established following intramuscular inoculation of the teat or intracutaneous inoculation of the mammary gland (Sarashina, pers. comm.). In the experiment of Tarry *et al.* (1978) infection was only established when infected *H. irritans* were used in combination with cutaneous damage to the teat, produced with a hypodermic needle.

It is unclear why the non-lactating mammary gland is most susceptible to infection. This might be due to the difficulty of slow growing bacteria establishing themselves within the gland when it is being flushed at milking time. Additionally the bacteria might be susceptible to intramammary defence mechanisms which are active in milk *e.g.* the lactoperoxidase system (Marshall *et al.*, 1986). Differences in oxygen availability in the actively secreting gland compared to the involuted gland may be important as may compositional differences in the secretion. *A. pyogenes* grows best in milk when the pH is > 7 and most *P. indolicus* strains are unable to grow once oxygen tension reaches 0.5%. The pH of the secretion of the non-lactating gland is usually > 7 and the presence of sulphydryl groups lowers redox potential and may stimulate *P. indolicus* directly or by antagonising the lactoperoxidase system. However these various influences have not been fully explored and demand further research.

DIAGNOSIS

Clinically, summer mastitis is readily diagnosed. The major limitations to early diagnosis and thus commencement of therapy are the methods of animal husbandry employed and the timing of cases. Non-lactating animals are usually not subjected to the close scrutiny given to lactating animals. They are often pastured some distance from the main farm site, even on adjacent farms or common pastures, and outbreaks of the disease occur at a time when there is considerable pressure on the farm because of harvest. The stock may be examined only by observation from a distance and consequently cases are not detected until marked signs of udder swelling or systemic disease are present. The affected animal is often found standing alone with a swollen teat which is sometimes heavily covered by flies. The affected gland rapidly becomes hard and indurated and the secretion purulent, foul-smelling and bloody. Recent data showed that the clinical diagnosis of summer mastitis made by the veterinarian or stockman was correct about 80% of the time (Hillerton *et al.*, 1986a). Confusing infections were predominantly *Str. uberis*, *Str. dysgalactiae* or *Staphylococcus aureus*. A foul smell to the secretion was regarded as an important diagnostic sign by veterinarians but there are cases, or stages within an infection, when no such odour is detected.

On this basis the need for improved accuracy of diagnosis might be questioned. However if 20% of suspected cases are wrongly diagnosed as summer mastitis and drastic action such as teat amputation or culling taken, when a more conservative approach might have been effective, then there are economic consequences of misdiagnosis.

It is unlikely that diagnosis based upon traditional bacteriological techniques will be of value. *A. pyogenes* cannot be reliably detected in < 48 h and *P. indolicus* may take several days to grow. Adequate selective anaerobic media to improve the isolation and identification of *P. indolicus* are lacking and would be advantageous. Nevertheless the delay is too great to be of practical, as opposed to scientific, value. More rapid diagnosis might be possible by gas liquid chromatography of the secretion to detect volatiles of diagnostic value. However such a technique requires a laboratory and expensive equipment. Perhaps a simple, cow-side test might subsequently be developed to identify the presence of particular compounds in the secretion. Assuming that *A. pyogenes* toxin is the most critical factor in the pathological changes of summer mastitis then an immunological test to detect the toxin, possibly by ELISA, might be useful and rapid. Alternatively since the secretion usually contains very high numbers of the bacteria (in contrast to many infections in lactating cows) a rapid test based on immunofluorescence might be applied.

EXPERIMENTAL STUDIES IN THE TRANSMISSION OF SUMMER MASTITIS

J.E. Hillerton, A.J. Bramley

Milking and Mastitis Centre,
AFRC Institute for Research on Animal Disease,
Compton, Berks, RG16 0NN, U.K.

ABSTRACT

Intramammary infusion of *Actinomyces pyogenes* or *Peptostreptococcus indolicus* causes clinical disease in the non-lactating bovine. The severity of the infection is greater when an inoculum of both organisms is used. Infection has resulted from contamination of teat skin with *A. pyogenes* but not *P. indolicus*. The fly, *Hydrotaea irritans*, was shown to contaminate the teat skin with bacteria but no infections resulted. However, the number of *A. pyogenes* presented to the teat skin by each fly was very low.

INTRODUCTION

Summer mastitis is a complex bacterial infection (Stuart *et al.*, 1951) and it is still unclear how, or in what sequence, the relevant pathogens, *Actinomyces pyogenes* and *Peptostreptococcus indolicus* invade the udder. Tarry *et al.* (1978) claimed that the fly, *Hydrotaea irritans*, could contaminate the teat of a supposedly healthy cow sufficiently for infections with a mixed flora, including the anaerobe, to occur within a few days. The following experiments using *A. pyogenes* and *P. indolicus* singly and in combination are part of a programme to elucidate the natural mechanism of transmission of summer mastitis.

EXPERIMENTAL

Infusion of 10^6-10^7 colony forming units (cfu) of *P. indolicus* 13/83 induced clinical mastitis in 77% of udder quarters of dry cows and heifers (Hillerton, 1985). The infections were mild, with limited systemic signs, were eliminated spontaneously within 14 days and did not persist into lactation.

Infusion of 3×10^5 cfu *A. pyogenes* 0367 into non-lactating glands resulted in clinical disease within 2 days in all 12 quarters used (Table 1). The infections persisted throughout the dry period and, although the animals were not severely ill, antibiotic therapy was considered necessary for 2 cows.

TABLE 1.   Effect of infusing 2 quarters of each of 6 dry cows with *A. pyogenes*.

	Days after infusion		
	2	4	7
Recovery of *A. pyogenes*	12/12	10/10	7/7
Clinical signs	10/12	5/6	6/7

In a further experiment *P. indolicus* infections were established in one quarter of each of 5 dry cows by inoculation of 3×10^7 cfu. This quarter and another uninfected quarter in each animal were then infused with 3×10^5 cfu *A. pyogenes*. *A. pyogenes* was subsequently recovered from all infused glands (Table 2). *P. indolicus* recovery was more intermittent; from 4/5 glands after 4 days and from the fifth gland after 7 days. Quarters infected only with *A. pyogenes* showed mild clinical disease and none required therapy. In contrast 3 animals having quarters with a mixed infection produced systemic signs after 4 days and were treated. A fourth animal subsequently required therapy.

TABLE 2.   Effect of superimposing *A. pyogenes* on an infection created by *P. indolicus*.

	Days after infusion		
	2	4	7
Recovery of *A. pyogenes*			
— *P. indolicus* quarters	5/5	5/5	2/2
— others	5/5	5/5	5/5
Recovery of *P. indolicus*	3/5	4/5	1/2

A second series of experiments involved applying *A. pyogenes* and *P. indolicus*, alone or in combination, to the teat surface. An undetermined inoculum from cultures grown for 18 h in cooked meat medium was applied to the teat orifice of pregnant heifers with a cotton wool swab. In some experiments cutaneous damage was created by pricking the skin of the swab site before contamination with a hypodermic needle. The damage was considered similar to that caused by biting flies and as used by Tarry *et al*. (1978).

Clinical infection of the mammary gland resulted twice with *A. pyogenes* being reisolated. Additionally *A. pyogenes* were twice recovered from mammary gland secretion when no clinical signs were apparent (Table 3). All 4 positive results occurred when *P. indolicus* were also present in the inoculum but the anaerobe was never recovered. Cutaneous damage was not necessary for infection to occur since 3 of the 4 infections, and both clinical cases, occurred in its absence.

It has been supposed that the natural mechanism of transmission involves contamination of the teats by flies. Hillerton and Thomas (1986) suggested that flies regurgitate the bacteria on to the teats and this has been further investigated. *H. irritans* were fed on blood containing 10^6 cfu *A. pyogenes* for 10 s only and then, after an interval of 2, 4 or 6 h, allowed to feed for 10 s on a sterile, second meal. The number of *A. pyogenes* introduced into the second meal was determined.

TABLE 3. Intramammary infection and mastitis following challenge of intact or damage teat skin with *A. pyogenes* (Ap) and/or *P. indolicus* (Pi).

	Bacteria only				Bacteria + damage		
	Control	Ap	Pi	Ap + Pi	Ap	Pi	Ap + Pi
No. of challenges	17	23	24	18	0	0	12
No. of clinical infections	0	0	0	2	0	0	0
No of recoveries	0	0	0	1	0	0	1

With a 2 h interval the subsequent meal was rarely contaminated although all flies used were shown to contain large numbers of *A. pyogenes* internally (Table 4). The number of subsequent meals contaminated increased with the interval between meals used. There was no difference between citrated blood and reconstituted milk as the second meal. However relatively few *A. pyogenes* were introduced by the fly. As flies have little need to regurgitate on a fully liquid meal, partly dried blood was later used. This was contaminated more frequently and with a tenfold increase in the number of *A. pyogenes* introduced. *P. indolicus* were also used in this experiment and recovered from the second meal.

TABLE 4. Recovery of *A. pyogenes* from a sterile second meal after infected *H. irritans* had been allowed to feed.

Exp.	Interval between meals	2 nd meal	No. +ve flies	$\bar{x}$ cfu *A. pyogenes*	No. *A. pyogenes* +ve flies used
1	2 h	citrated blood	0	0	10
2	2 h	citrated blood	1	4	5
	2 h	milk	2	9	5
	4 h	citrated blood	2	4	5
	4 h	milk	2	2	5
	6 h	citrated blood	4	19	5
	6 h	milk	4	6	5
3	2 h	partly dried blood	10	623	10
	6 h	partly dried blood	7	530	7

Using a similar procedure the infected flies were then presented to undamaged teats of pregnant heifers for their second meal. All teats were swabbed before and after 10 flies per teat were allowed access for 30 min. All flies carried *A. pyogenes* and *P. indolicus*. On only 1/12 exposures was *A. pyogenes* recovered, equivalent to 240 cfu on the teat, a similar number to that introduced to sterile blood by the fly feeding. On this occasion although 10 flies were exposed to the teat only one could be proven to have fed whilst on the teat.

CONCLUSIONS

Infection with *A. pyogenes* or *P. indolicus* can produce clinical disease in the the non-lactating mammary gland but combined infection leads to clinically more severe disease.

External contamination of the teat with *A. pyogenes* causes intramammary infection, presumably by the bacteria passing through the teat duct. *P. indolicus* appears unable to invade the gland by the same route.

Infected *H. irritans* can contaminate teat skin by regurgitation but only with a few hundred cfu *A. pyogenes*. It remains to be proven if so few bacteria are sufficient to induce intramammary infection.

A STUDY OF THE AETIOLOGY OF SUMMER MASTITIS USING EXPERIMENTAL INFECTIONS

U. Vecht, H.J. Wisselink and A.M. Ham-Hoffies

Central Veterinary Institute,
P.O. Box 65, 8200 AB Lelystad, The Netherlands

ABSTRACT

A number of bacterial species are commonly associated with summer mastitis, such as *Corynebacterium pyogenes, Peptococcus indolicus* and *Fusobacterium necrophorum*. In order to study the aetiology of this disease 16 dry heifers were inoculated via the teat canal with monocultures and various combinations of these three species. Combinations of *Corynebacterium pyogenes* and *Peptococcus indolicus*, with or without *Fusobacterium necrophorum*, and the combination *Peptococcus indolicus* with *Fusobacterium necrophorum* resulted in a clinically acute purulent mastitis, typical for summer mastitis. All infected quarters yielded positive isolations within 5 days of infusion.

Inocula with bacterial numbers of *circ.* 6×10^8 C.F.U. of *Corynebacterium pyogenes* and *Peptococcus indolicus* resulted in the typical clinical symptoms within 24 hours, positive isolations within 3 days and the typical summer mastitis secretion 5 days after inoculation. Serum iron, zinc and haematological values were measured at four hour intervals after experimental infection. Serum iron showed an average decrease from 27 μmol/L to 13 μmol/L, and serum zinc from 15 μmol/L to 11 μmol/L 24 hours after inoculation. Neutrophil granulocytes rose from values averaging 2.93×10^9/L to 6.94×10^9/L. These animals showed fever. Similar results were obtained with the group inoculated with all three species.

The observed changes in trace metals, neutrophils and body temperature are characteristic for an early host response to infection, probably mediated by members of the interleukine-1 family.

INTRODUCTION

A number of bacterial species are commonly associated with summer mastitis such as: *Corynebacterium pyogenes, Peptococcus indolicus, Streptococcus dysgalactiae*, an unnamed microaerophilic cocci and *Bacteroides* spp. The aetiology of summer mastitis, with regard to the many species which may be involved, is still unclear (Tolle *et al.*, 1983). *C. pyogenes* is usually isolated in combination with non-sporulating obligate anaerobic bacteria (OAB). Sometimes these OAB are found in higher frequency than *C. pyogenes* (Sorensen, 1974; Schwan *et al.*, 1979; Greeff *et al.*, 1983). Sometimes OAB, *e.g. Fusobacterium necrophorum*, are isolated as the only pathogens from mastitic udders (Shinjo, 1983; McGillivery, 1984).

In the Netherlands the most frequently isolated microorganisms from cases suspected of summer mastitis in 1984 and 1985 were *Corynebacterium pyogenes* (37%), *Peptococcus indolicus* (33%) and *Fusobacterium necrophorum* (22%). (Vecht *et al.*, 1986). Hence, experimental infections with various combinations of these three species were carried out in order to study the aetiology of summer mastitis.

MATERIAL AND METHODS

Bacterial strains of *C. pyogenes, P. indolicus* and *F. necrophorum* were primarily isolated from field cases of summer mastitis. Storage was in Horni-Brook medium at −70°C. Inocula were prepared by separate incubation of each strain in 20 ml Brain Heart Infusion (BHI) broth supplemented with cysteine, hemin and vit K_1. Incubation at 37°C in an anaerobic glovebox lasted 24 hrs. for *C. pyogenes* and 18 hrs. for *P. indolicus* and *F. necrophorum*. Cultures were reincubated by adding the 20 ml volume to 80 ml fresh BHI suppl. broth: incubation lasted 24 hrs. for *C. pyogenes* and 3 hrs. for *P. indolicus* and *F. necrophorum*. Purity was checked on solid media (BHI suppl. agar with 6% horse blood). Cultures were centrifuged at 1000 Fg, and resuspended in BHI (suppl.) broth. Using spectrophotometer extinction values inocula were prepared as close as possible to 5×10^8 CFU.

Two experiments were carried out:

In experiment 1, eight one year old heifers were inoculated via the teat canal with the four combinations of strains listed in Table 1. Two animals were used per combination, two udder quarters being infused in each animal.

In experiment 2, two groups of four heifers, each one year of age, were infected via the teat canal with a combination of *C. pyogenes* and *P. indolicus*, and with *C. pyogenes, P. indolicus* and *F. necrophorum*. Inoculum size was 6.1×10^8 for *C. pyogenes*, 6.2×10^8 for *P. indolicus* and 3.2×10^9 for *F. necrophorum*. Two quarters per animal were infused.

Experimental animals were clinically examined twice daily. Blood and serum samples were taken at four hour intervals during the first 24 hours after infection and daily thereafter. Secretion samples for bacteriology were sampled daily, only when the quarters showed clear clinical symptoms.

Serum iron concentrations were determined by centrifugal analysis (Flexigen[®]) using Ferrozinc Reagent[®][1]. Serum zinc levels were analysed using atomic absorption. Total leucocyte counts in EDTA blood were made with a conducting counter (Contraves[®])[2]. Neutrophil counts were calculated from the total counts and the differential counts on smears. Quarter samples were cultured on BHI suppl. agar with 6% horse blood and in deoxygenated serum broth. Media were incubated anaerobically at 37°C and the agar checked for growth every 48 hrs. for 5 days. After five days of incubation, the serum broth was subcultured on the BHI agar and grown anaerobically for another 5 day period. Identification was according to standard procedures (Holdeman *et al.*, 1977 and Cowan and Steel, 1974).

RESULTS

Experiment 1. The four different combinations of bacterial species, with inoculum

[1] Gemini, Electro-nucleonics Inc. Fairfield N.Y., U.S.A.
[2] Contraves A.G. Zurich, Switzerland.

size (total number of CFU) and clinical results are given in Table I.

TABLE I.   Clinical results after intramammary infection with 4 inocula.

Inoculum	C.F.U.		Swelling quarter, with pain and fever					
		day	1	2	3	4	5	6
1. *C. pyogenes*	3.2×10^7		−	−	−	−	−	−
2. *P. indolicus*	3.6×10^7		−	−	−	±*	±*	±*
3. *P. indolicus* +	8.0×10^6		±	±	+	++	+++	+++
F. necrophorum	3.3×10^6							
4. *C. pyogenes* +	3.2×10^7		±	+	++	++	+++	+++
P. indolicus	3.6×10^7							

* in one quarter only, no raise in body temperature.

Inoculation with only *C. pyogenes* did not result in inflammation. Inoculation with *P. indolicus* in monoculture resulted in only one inflamed quarter out of 4 infusions. Findings were not typical for summer mastitis: moderate swelling with no fever or other general symptoms. With the combinations *P. indolicus* and *F. necrophorum* (combination nr. 3) and also with *C. pyogenes* together with *P. indolicus* (combination nr. 4) clinical symptoms which were typical for summer mastitis were observed within 3 days of infusion. The combination of *P. indolicus* with *F. necrophorum* had an even smaller inoculum size (see Table I) than the other infusions. Clinical symptoms consisted of swelling, hardness, pain and raised temperature of the infused quarter locally and fever and lack of appetite systemically.

Positive isolations for all infusions were found within 5 days of inoculation. Earlier recovery of bacteria was not feasible since no secretions could be sampled. The typical secretion for summer mastitis i.e. yellow-green pus with foul odour was only seen with combinations nr. 3 and 4 after twelve and five days of infection respectively.

Experiment 2. Combinations of both *C. pyogenes, P. indolicus* (group 1) and *C. pyogenes, P. indolicus, F. necrophorum* (group 2) with the larger inoculum size resulted in clinical symptoms typical for summer mastitis in both groups of heifers within 24 hrs. of inoculation. Bacteriology was positive for all animals within three days and remained so during the experiment. Each bacterial species which had been inoculated could be recovered daily. The typical summer mastitis secretion was observed after 5 days. Four days after infection, body temperatures had returned to normal. Clinical symptoms in all 8 animals were remarkably uniform: *i.e.* swelling, hardness, oedema, pain and raised temperature of the infused quarter locally and fever with lack of appetite systemically. One animal (group 1) showed oedema in the hind legs. No other clinical differences between group 1 and 2 could be observed.

Serum iron, zinc and neutrophil leucocyte counts were measured from blood samples collected at four hour intervals during the first 24 hours after infection and daily before and after that period. These clinical pathology and haematology results are depicted in Figure 1 (serum iron), Figure 2 (serum zinc) and Figure 3 (neutrophil leucocyte count).

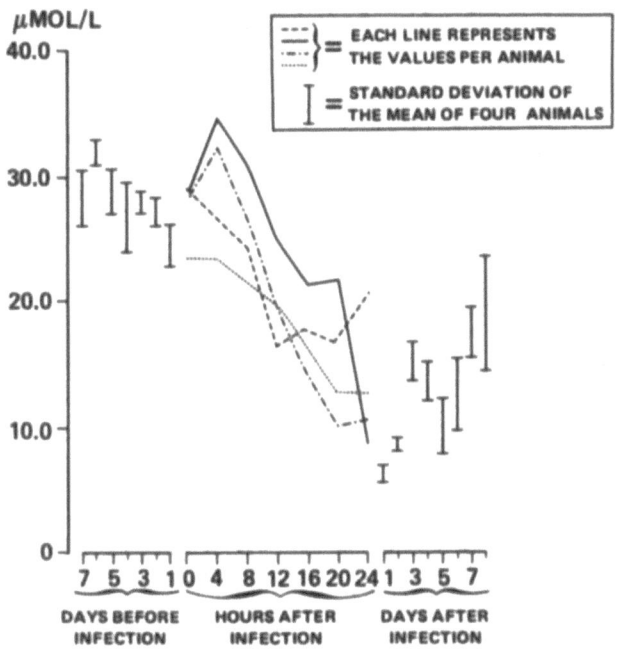

Figure 1. Clinical Pathology: Serum iron values of four heifers after experimental infection with *C. pyogenes* and *P. indolicus* (6.1×10^8 : 6.2×10^8 C.F.U.)

Serum iron showed an average decrease from 27 μmol/L (s.d. 2.6) to 13 μmol/L (s.d. 5.2) 24 hrs. after inoculation. Serum zinc decreased from an average of 15 μmol/L (s.d. 3.7) to 11 μmol/L 24 hrs. after inoculation. Neutrophil leucocyte numbers rose from values averaging 2.93×10^9/L to 6.9×10^9/L. Similar results were obtained with the four heifers inoculated with *C. pyogenes, P. indolicus* and *F. necrophorum.*

94

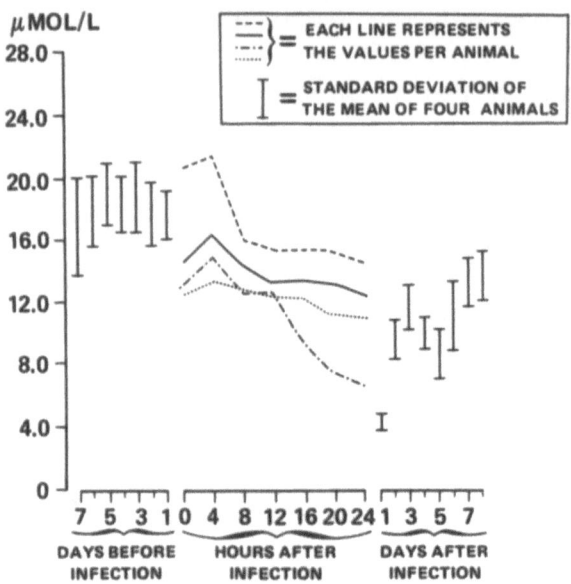

Figure 2. Clinical Pathology: Serum zinc (Zn) values of four heifers after experimental infection with *C. pyogenes* and *P. indolicus* (6.1 x 10^8 :6.2 x 10^8 C.F.U.)

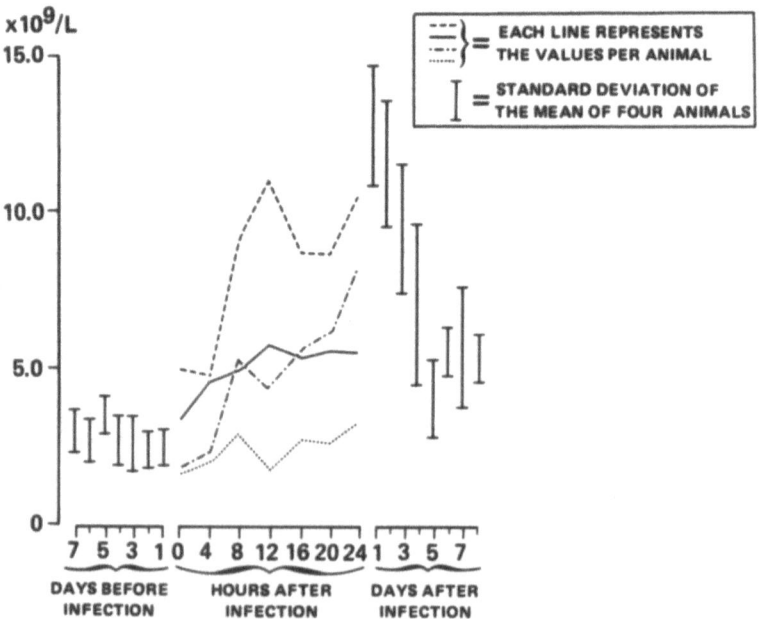

Figure 3. Haematology: neutrophil leucocyte counts of four heifers after experimental infection with *C. pyogenes* and *P. indolicus* (6.1 x 10^8 :6.2 x 10^8 C.F.U.)

DISCUSSION

It appeared that experimental infection with monocultures of C. pyogenes at the used dosages could not induce acute mastitis in heifers. With P. indolicus, only mild symptoms were observed, which is in agreement with earlier observations by Hillerton (1985). Effects appeared dose dependent as the infection with combinations of C. pyogenes and P. indolicus with CFU's of circ. 6×10^8 resulted in severe clinical symptoms within 24 hours. Less severe effects, only 3 days after infection were observed when inocula with lower numbers of bacteria (circ. 3×10^7) were used. Earlier experiments with inocula of C. pyogenes combined with P. indolicus with CFU of circ. 10^4 did not result in establishment of infection at all.

The combination of P. indolicus with F. necrophorum resulted in acute purulent mastitis clinically indistinguishable from summer mastitis. In fact it appeared that at the used dosage, the combination of P. indolicus with F. necrophorum (CFU $8.0 \times 10^6 : 3.3 \times 10^6$) did result in inflammation while the combination C. pyogenes + P. indolicus (CFU $1.5 \times 10^7 : 3.3 \times 10^6$) with a comparable bacterial count failed to do so. This supports our earlier observations that establishment of infection is dose dependant and that symptoms typical for summer mastitis can be the consequence of infection by a combination of OAB without C. pyogenes.

The typical summer mastitis secretion of a yellow green pus with foul odour is only seen several days after infection. Depending on the constitution and dosage of infection this varied from 5 to 12 days, which could hinder rapid diagnosis under field conditions.

In accordance with earlier studies (Sorensen, 1972), it appeared that a combination of C. pyogenes with OAB leads to severe mastitis in the dry udder.

Besides clinical and bacteriological variables, the disease was also studied using haematology and clinical chemistry. If an animal is exposed to an exogenous insult it responds e.g. with a series of dramatic changes in metabolic and immunological functions. Most of these changes are observed within hours of the onset of infection or inflammation. Therefore, these non-specific host responses are termed the "acute-phase reaction". The most fundamental event in the initiation of this reaction is the production of mediator molecules called the interleukin-1 family, polypeptides which induce clinical, haemotological and chemical changes of the acute phase response (van Miert, 1986). Interleukin-1 (IL-1) is a product of circulating phagocytic cells and tissue macrophages in liver, spleen and respiratory tract. A good clinical example to illustrate the effect of IL-1 on the host has been shown in cows with acute coliform mastitis (Verheijden et al., 1983). Local effects of IL-1 in the surrounding tissues of the udder include: cellular infiltration, hyperaemia, secretion of lactoferrin and transferrin in the milk, which are active against mastitis pathogens. General effects of IL-1 polypeptides include an increase in number and immaturity of circulating neutrophils, hypozincaemia, hypoferraemia and induction of fever. Such changes were observed in this study, indicating that cattle infected with pathogens causing summer mastitis show this early host response to infection. This could prove an excellent tool to monitor the progression of the disease or for investigating the efficacy of prophylactic and, or curative measures.

When using inocula with higher bacterial counts we could not find any differences in clinical results, aspect of secretion, recovery time of inoculated organisms from secretion, trace minerals in serum and haematologic values between the groups infected with *C. pyogenes* and *P. indolicus* and the group with *C. pyogenes, P. indolicus* and *F. necrophorum*.

CONCLUSIONS

Experimental infection with *P. indolicus* and *F. necrophorum* can produce clinical symptoms typical for summer mastitis. The effect of experimental infection is dose dependent.

Experimental infection of *C. pyogenes* and *P. indolicus* with *circ.* 6×10^8 CFU results *e.q.* in rapid decrease in serum iron and zinc, increase in neutrophil counts and fever within 24 hours of inoculation. Such changes are characteristic for an acute phase response to infection which may be mediated by interleukin-1 polypeptides. These parameters are suitable for monitoring the progression of summer mastitis after infection.

Experimental infection both with combinations of *C. pyogenes, P. indolicus* and *F. necrophorum* and with *C. pyogenes* and *P. indolucus* produces the same clinical, pathological, bacteriological and haematological effects.

ACKNOWLEDGEMENTS

We wish to thank the National Animal Health Committee for supporting the research.

REFERENCES

Bean, C.W., Miller, W.T. and Heishman, J.O. 1943. A note on *Corynebacterium pyogenes* as the cause of bovine mastitis. J. A. V. M. A., **103**, 200-202.

Bramley, A.J., Hillerton, J.E., Higgs, T.M. and Hogben, E.M. 1985. The carriage of summer mastitis pathogens by muscid flies. Br. vet. J., **141**, 618-627.

Cowan, S.T. and Steel, K.J. 1974. Manual for the identification of medical bacteria. Cambridge University Press, Cambridge, 238 pp.

Du Preez, J.H., Greef, A.S. and Eksteen, N. 1981. Isolation and significance of anaerobic bacteria isolated from cases of bovine mastitis. Ond. J. vet. Res., **48**, 123-126.

Egan, J. 1985. Evidence of *Corynebacterium pyogenes* as a secondary pathogen in mastitis in lactating cows. Kiel. Milch. Forschung., **37**, 585-588.

Gibbs, H.A. 1986. Mycoplasma mastitis outbreak. Vet. Rec., **118**, 466.

Greeff, A.S., Du Preez, J.H. and de Beer, Maria. 1983. The frequency and some characteristics of anaerobic bacteria isolated from various forms of bovine mastitis. J. of the S.A. Vet. Ass., **1**, 25-28.

Hansen, J.V. and Nielsen, S.A. 1983. Summer Mastitis. Proc. Heifer Mastitis Seminar, Stockholm-Helsinki. Svensk Husdjurrskotsel ek for.

Hillerton, J.E. 1985a. Infection of lactating and dry cows with *Peptococcus indolicus*, Proc. IDF Seminar, Progress in the Control of Bovine Mastitis, Kiel 21-24 May, 601-604.

Hillerton, J.E. 1985b. Infection of lactating and dry cows with *Peptococcus indolicus*. Kiel. Milch. Forschung., **37**, 601-604.

Hillerton, J.E., Bramley, A.J. and Broom, D.M. 1983. *Hydrotaea irritans* and summer mastitis in calves. Vet. Rec., **113**, 88.

Hillerton, J.E., Bramley, A.J. and Broom, D.M. 1984. The distribution of five species of flies (Diptera: Muscidae) over the bodies of dairy heifers in England. Bull. ent. Res., **74**, 113-119.

Hillerton, J.E., Bramley, A.J. and Watson, C.A. 1986a. Epidemiology of summer mastitis: a survey of clinical cases. Br. vet. J., (in press).

Hillerton, J.E., Morant, S.V. and Harris, J.A. 1986b. Control of Muscidae on cattle by flucythrinate ear tags, the behaviour of these flies on cattle and the effects of fly-dislodging behaviour. Entomol. exp. appl., **41**, 213-218.

Hillerton, J.E. and Thomas, G. 1986. Transmission of summer mastitis by flies. Abs. First Int. Cong. Dipterology, (Ed. B. Darvas and L. Papp) Budapest. p. 95.

Holdeman, L.V., Cato, E.P. and Moore, W.E.C. 1977. Anaerobe Laboratory Manual 4th ed. Virginia Polytechnic Institute and State University, Blacksburg, Virginia.

Jorgensen, K.L. 1937. Mastitis caused by mixed infection with *Corynebacterium pyogenes* and anaerobic microccocci. Maanedsskr. Dyrlaeg., **49**, 113-119.

Marshall, V.M., Cole, W.M. and Bramley, A.J. 1986. Influence of the lactoperoxidase system on the susceptibility of the udder to *Streptococcus uberis* infection. J. Dairy Res., (in press).

McGillivery, D.J. 1984. Isolation of *Fusobacterium necrophorum* from a case of bovine mastitis. Austr. Vet. J., **61** (10), 325.

Munch-Petersen, E. 1938. Bovine mastitis. Survey of the literature to the end of 1935. Imp. Bur. Animal Hlth. Weybridge.

Robinson, J. and Luff, M.L. 1979. Population estimates and dispersal of *Hydrotaea irritans*. Fallén. Ecol. Entomol., **4**, 289-296.

Schwan, O., Nord, C.E. and Holmberg, O. 1979. Biochemical characterization of unidentified microaerophilic cocci isolated from heifer mastitis and dry cow mastitis. J. Clin. Microb., **10**, 622-627.

Shinjo, T. 1983. *Fusobacterium necrophorum* isolated from a hepatic abscess and isolated from mastitic udder secretions in a heifer. Ann. Microbiol. Inst. Pasteur, **134 B**, 401-409.

Sorensen, G. Hoi. 1972. Sommer mastis eksperimentelt fremkaldt hos juvenile kvier. Nord. Vet. Med., **24**, 247-258.

Sorensen, G. Hoi. 1974. Studies on the aetiology and transmission of summer mastitis, Nord. Vet. Med., **26**, 122-132.

Sorensen, G. Hoi. 1976. Studies on the occurrence of *Peptococcus indolicus* and *Corynebacterium pyogenes* in apparently healthy cows. Act. Vet. Scand., **17**, 15-24.

Sorensen, G. Hoi. 1978. Bacteriological examination of summer mastitis secretions. The demonstration of Bacteroidaceae. Nord. Vet. Med., **30**, 199-204.

Sorensen, G. Hoi. 1980. Comparative studies of *Corynebacterium pyogenes* toxin formation in monocultures and mixed cultures. (The demonstration of a stimulating effect of *P. indolicus* and Stuart-Schwan cocci). Act. Vet. Scand., **21**, 438-447.

Stuart, P., Buntain, D. and Langridge, R.G. 1951. Bacteriological examination of secretions from cases of summer mastitis and experimental infection of non-lactating bovine udders. Vet. Rec., **63**, 451-453.

Tarry, D.W., Wilson, C.D. and Stuart, P. 1978. The headfly *Hydrotaea irritans* and summer mastitis infection. Vet. Rec., **102**, 91.

Tolle, A., Franke, V. and Reichmuth, J. 1983. Zur *C. pyogenes*-Mastitis: Bakteriologische Aspecte. Dtsch. tierärztl. Wschr., **90**, 256-260.

Tolle, A. and Reichmuth, J. 1985. Summer mastitis. Kiel. Milch. Forschung., **37**, 575-584.

Van Miert, A.S.J.P.A.M. 1986. Inflammation and febrile conditions: the role of Interleukin-I. Proc. IVth Int. Symp. of Veterinary Laboratory Diagnosticians, June 2-6, 1986, pp. 122-130.

Vecht, U., Wisselink, H.J., Sol, J. and Van den Bogaard, A.E.J.M. 1986. The bacteriological constitution of Dutch summer mastitis cases. Proc. C.E.C. Workshop Summer mastitis, 23-24 October, Lelystad, The Netherlands.

Verheijden, J.H.M., Van Miert, A.S.J.P.A.M., Schotman, A.J.H. and Van Duin, C.T.M. 1983. Pathophysiological aspects of *E. coli* mastitis in Ruminants. Veterinary Research Communications, **7**, 229-236.

Wright, C.L. and Titchener, R.N. 1977. Infection of the sheep headfly, *Hydrotaea irritans*, with bacterial isolates from field cases of summer mastitis. Vet. Rec., **101**, 426.

DISCUSSION

The discussion following the aetiology/pathogenesis session dealt mainly with two aspects:

1. bacteria: their interactions, virulence and mode of invasion.
2. the host: "triggering" mechanisms, predisposing infection, non-specific host response.

The mode of invasion was discussed in the context of the experimental infections which have been carried out. In Denmark the hypothesis is that flies only deposit bacteria on the teat and that other triggering mechanisms are necessary to cause infection. Such mechanisms could include dropping out of the plug, wounds, injuries by other dipterans such as *Haematobia irritans, Stomoxys calcitrans,* biting midges and blackflies. This is the reason why the teat plug is deliberately kept intact when experimental infections are carried out in the U.K. The bacteria deposited by the flies could be recovered in 1/12 of the cases. In trying to mimic wounds by biting insects, hypodermic needles were used, following by "painting" the teats with bacterial mixtures. This resulted in inflammation. An attempt in Holland to imitate the effect of biting flies using needles and dipping with high number of bacteria failed to produce disease. It was considered important that for these infections with anaerobic bacteria, media with reduced oxygen tension are used, such as cooked meat medium.

In considering aetiology it was observed in the U.K., that *Peptococcus indolicus* could be recovered from secretions of experimental animals which were not inoculated with these bacteria. On one occasion micro-aerophilic cocci were also recovered. In both the U.K. and the Netherlands it was observed that the dry udder secretion of apparently healthy cows is often contaminated with bacteria. Pathogens such as *S. aureus* and *P. indolicus* can be isolated from such animals. Another source of anaerobes could be the teat canal. In South Africa (du Preez) many species of anaerobes are regularly isolated from the keratine layer within the teat. Keratine with its mechanical and bactericidal properties is part of the defence of the udder against infection. Hence, when such bacteria are recovered, it is difficult to assess whether the animal concerned is successfully defending itself against an infection or whether it is going to suffer from infection (bacteria are ascending).

The experimental infection in Holland where the typical symptoms of summer mastitis were produced without *C. pyogenes* being inoculated could be important for a better understanding of the aetiology. In the U.K. and in Holland infections with *C. pyogenes* alone produced only mild local signs or no inflammation at all. This indicates that when *C. pyogenes* is not found in field cases one should not assume too lightly that *C. pyogenes* is "missed". It also suggests that we still know too little of the aetiology of summer mastitis: the sequence of invasion, colonization and inflammation by various species deserve more study. Furthermore, there is still much unknown about the virulence of strains within species, and the interaction of different species.

A new finding in the pathogenesis was the observed non-specific host response. Dutch experimental infections showed the typical increase in neutrophilic leucocytes together with the decrease in blood, iron and zinc levels and the presence of fever. The extant theory is that Interleukin 1 (IL1) stimulates the secretion of antimicrobial, cationic proteins (lacto-ferrin, transferrin). It has been shown that human IL1 causes neutrophils to release specific granulae contents including lactoferrin. The lactoferrin iron complex is hence deposited in the reticulo-endothelial system. This partly explains the hypoferraemia. It is suggested that this phenomenon together with fever and neutrophilia acts as a co-ordinated, non-specific host response.

It was speculated that stress caused by poor nutrition could act as a predisposing factor in bacterial infection. The relation stress-virulence factors and aetiology deserves further study.

4. TRANSMISSION OF THE DISEASE

Chairmen G. Thomas & B. Overgaard Nielsen

CATTLE FLIES AND THE TRANSMISSION OF SUMMER MASTITIS

G. Thomas

Dept. of Parasitology, Central Veterinary Institute,
Postbox 65, 8200 AB Lelystad, The Netherlands.
Dept. of Animal Physiology, University of Groningen, The Netherlands.

ABSTRACT

A review is made of the evidence underlying the two hypotheses formulated to explain the cause of summer mastitis epidemics. One of these supposes an endogenous source of bacteria and the occurrence of clinical disease when this is triggered by a season specific triggering mechanism. The alternative hypothesis proposes that summer mastitis is a vector transmitted disease and that 1 of the 40-50 cattle fly species, *viz., Hydrotaea irritans* is the principle vector. Evidence supporting the latter hypothesis includes temporal and spatial factors, fly behaviour, the effect of vector control measures, presence of the bacteria in the fly and successful artificial and actual transmission experiments.

INTRODUCTION

Heifer or summer mastitis is an acute, suppurative mastitis which occurs in calves, heifers and non-lactating cows. The infection has a complex aetiology and a number of bacterial species may be isolated from the highly purulent secretion including *Corynebacterium pyogenes*, a range of OAB including *Peptococcus indolicus*, often a Gram positive microaerophilic coccus, and *Streptococcus dysgalactiae* (Stuart *et al.*, 1951; Sorensen, 1974, 1978). Although infections caused by members of this bacterial complex are common the whole year round, explosive outbreaks of the disease can occur in the months of July, August and September in the temperate palaearctic region when animals are at pasture. As a consequence, this form of mastitis in non-lactating cattle is frequently referred to as summer mastitis. Whether or not summer mastitis may be considered a distinct disease in bacteriological, aetiological or pathenogenic terms is arguable. However, the incidence pattern of the summer peak strongly suggests that a different, but not necessarily mutually exclusive, set of epidemiological variables are involved at this season of the year. A considerable amount of correlative evidence has been proposed indicating that a vector transmission mechanism is involved. Only one alternative hypothesis has been suggested to explain the summer peak. This assumes the presence of an endogenous infection, but obviously a season specific triggering mechanism is also required to explain the epidemiological pattern.

The main aim of this paper is to review the evidence underlying the hypotheses formulated with respect to the causality of summer mastitis.

THE ENDOGENOUS HYPOTHESIS

Lovell (1943, 1945) was one of the first researchers to suggest that the ultimate cause of summer mastitis infections was a latent, endogenous source of bacteria and that clinical disease only appears when initiated or triggered by one or another proximate factor. He pointed to the fact that *C. pyogenes* was frequently present in the mucous membranes of apparently healthy cattle, sheep and goats. Ochi and Zaizen (in Lovell, 1943) and Francis (1941) for example, recovered this bacterium from mucous and urine in a large percentage of the normally healthy cattle examined. Positive sites included the mucous membranes of the mouth, nose, vagina and the tonsils. Later work by Sorensen (1976) not only confirmed the regular presence of latent *C. pyogenes* infection in apparently healthy cattle but also demonstrated that this was true for the OAB *Peptococcus indolicus*. He found this bacterium in the vagina, nasal cavity and tonsils at percentages of $\sim$ 23, 10 and 55 of respectively in the cows examined and 73% in the tonsils of young bulls. Natterman and Horsch (1976) suggested that establishment of the bacteria in udder tissue may occur from the above sites as a consequence of sucking behaviour and/or via a lymphohaematogenic route of infection. Spread of the bacteria through the cattle population has been attributed to transmission by the bull (McEwen, 1942) but is has also been suggested that flies may spread the infection from cow to cow (Anon., 1942; Campbell, 1941). Madsen *et al.* (1986) carried out a study on incidence of *C. pyogenes* and *P. indolicus* contamination of the udder epidermis on healthy heifers as a function of time and found that during winter and spring in the stall between 18 and 19% of the population was affected. This value decreased to almost zero after turn-out and remained low until mid-summer when it rose steeply to 70% or so. The percentage slowly decreased again during autumn reaching a level of approximately 20% by the following winter. The authors pointed out that the form of the summer peak in incidence corresponded closely to the population density curve for *Hydrotaea irritans*, the fly most suspected as a carrier of summer mastitis pathogens.

No systematic research has been carried out to identify the proximate aetiological factors which have been hypothesised as being involved in initiating or triggering a clinical infection. Lovell (1943, 1945) suggested that some other bacterial and viral infections or injury may stimulate a latent *C. pyogenes* infection into activity. Moreover, he indicated that the irritation set up by flies may also be a factor in the aetiology. Heavy fly pestation can certainly lead to stress of the host and a large body of literature now exists demonstrating that stress can act negatively on the immune system (see *e.g.* Stein *et al.*, 1985) and udder health (Giesecke, 1985). Finally, decrease in condition of the host as grazing quality deteriorates over the summer should also be taken into consideration as essential nutrient element deficiencies or imbalances of several elements can lead to detrimental effects on animal health and resistance to pathogens and parasites *etc* (see *e.g.* Horvath and Reid, 1984).

THE VECTOR TRANSMISSION HYPOTHESIS

The hypothesis that summer mastitis is a fly vector transmitted disease is a relatively old one (Campbell, 1941; Anon., 1942). Of the 40 to 50 species commonly found on cattle in northern Europe (see Liebisch and Overgaard Nielsen, this section), the females of one species in particular are considered to be most likely involved in the transmission of the disease. This species is the haematophagous, non-biting muscid *Hydrotaea irritans*. According to Tarry (1975), the females of this species require up to 9 protein meals for ovarian maturation and these they obtain from mammalian hosts. The major arguments are as follows:

1. Temporal factors

Many authors have pointed to the fact that the start of the summer mastitis season is synchronous with the emergence of *H. irritans* and moreover, that the annual population dynamics curve for this species fits the seasonal summer mastitis incidence curve almost exactly (see Bramley, sect. 3; Hansen and Nielsen, 1983). In many of the other common cattle visiting Diptera, peak population levels in the vicinity of cattle are later: *Stomoxys calcitrans, Haematobosca (Haematobia) stimulans, Haematobia (Lyperosia) irritans*. Some are earlier: *Hydrotaea meteorica, Haematopota* spec., Simuliidae, or non-coincidental: *Hydrotaea albipuncta, Morellia simplex* (Ball, 1984; Liebisch, this section). As peak fly activity might rationally be expected to occur earlier in lower latitudes than in more northern ones this should be accompanied by a comparable shift in peak incidence of the disease. There are data indicating that the latter does indeed occur. In the province of Limburg in the Netherlands peak incidences occur in early July (Saes, 1970) whereas in Denmark this is in August (Nansen, 1985). Unfortunately, simultaneous, quantitative fly dynamics data are lacking in respect to temporal shifts in peak with latitude.

2. Spatial factors

All major summer mastitis areas in northern Europe are overlapped by the macro-geographic distribution of *H. irritans*. Skidmore (1985) states that the distribution of this species is palaeoarctic, extending from the west of Britain to northern Greece and from Sweden to southern Spain and even Israel. The spatial coincidence between high incidence summer mastitis areas and areas with a high *H. irritans* density is also found at the micro-geographical level. Hansen and Nielsen (1983) and Madsen *et al.* (1986) found a positive relation between local fly density and disease incidence.

3. Fly behaviour

Summer mastitis outbreaks tend to occur during specific climatic conditions *e.g.* Olesen *et al.* (1985) found a relation between increased incidence in summer mastitis and an immediately foregoing 10 day period of high air temperature and low wind velocity. Other researchers have found that the same climatic conditions favour high *H. irritans* activity (Nielsen *et al.*, 1985c). High air temperature and humidity increased the visitation rate of *H. irritans* to its cattle host whereas an increase in wind speed reduced this.

It is reasonable to assume that one requirement for a vector of summer mastitis is that it makes frequent contact with the infection site on the host. As far as *H. irritans* is concerned, it feeds copiously on udder originating fluids (Thomas *et al.*, 1985) and, moreover, it does forage regularly on the udder (Nielsen *et al.*, 1985b). This is particularly true when its potential as a feeding site is increased by the presence of wounds caused by biting flies such as some species of biting midges (Ceratopogonidae), blackflies (Simuliidae), mosquitoes (Culicidae) and horseflies (Tabanidae).

4. Vector control measures

One of the crucial arguments supporting the hypothesis that summer mastitis is a fly vector transmitted disease is the fact that control of insects with insecticide or other fly prevention measures can lead to large reduction in summer mastitis incidence. Aehnelt (1955), using a long acting contact insecticide, obtained a difference of 0.7 and 9.4% incidence in treated and non-treated herds respectively. Similar reduction in summer mastitis incidence has been found by numerous other workers. Marshall (1981) on the other hand, although achieving considerable reduction in fly numbers after using a pour-on, only found differences of 2.05 and 2.55% incidence in treated and non-treated animals respectively. One major difference between the two applications was that Aehnelt paid particular attention to spraying the udder and even used three times as high concentrations in this region. This suggests that control of udder visiting flies is the crucial element. This is supported by the results of some Danish experiments where 60 to 100% reduction in incidence was obtained by simply preventing flies having access to the teat by using micropore plaster bandages (Hansen and Nielsen, 1983). This latter experiment may also have a further implication. As the method only prevents access to the teat surface, its effect on fly species and numbers on the cattle host will be low and should not have a major impact on fly-caused host stress, thus weakening the possible involvement of this factor as a role in the aetiology of summer mastitis.

5. Bacteriological investigations of potential vectors

In hypothesising the involvement of a fly in the transmission of summer mastitis it is essential to demonstrate that the causative pathogens can be carried by the potential vector. Bahr (1955) was the first researcher to examine field caught flies for the presence of *C. pyogenes* and found that 1.5-2% of the *H. irritans* he examined to contain this bacterium. Recoveries were only obtained from the interior of the fly and not from the outer surface. Since then two other studies have been carried out to examine cattle flies for summer mastitis pathogens. Their results are summarised in Table 1.

TABLE 1. Pathogens isolated from cattle flies. Data taken from Sorensen, 1974;
Bramley *et al.*, 1985.

Positive species	Sorensen		Bramley *et al.*	
	N. flies examined	% positives	N. flies examined	% positives
H. irritans	260	6.9	825	3.3
H. meteorica	—	—	4	25.0
Ha. irritans	—	—	1044	0.2
S. calcitrans	—	—	98	1.0
M. autumnalis	—	—	364	0.6
Simulium spp.	130	2.3	—	—
Culicoides spp.	114	0.9	—	—
Others	60	0.0	195	0.0

As far as known summer mastitis pathogens are concerned, Sorensen recovered *C. pyogenes, P. indolicus* and *Str. dysgalactiae* from *H. irritans, C. pyogenes* and *P. indolicus* from *Simulium* spp. and only *C. pyogenes* from *Culicoides* spp. In Bramley *et al.*'s findings the three above mentioned bacteria were all found in *H. irritans* and *H. meteorica, C. pyogenes* and *Str. uberis* in *M. autumnalis* and the remaining fly species only contained *S. aureus*. Wright and Titchener (1977) used a different approach to determine if *H. irritans* could carry summer mastitis pathogens. They artificially infected flies with monocultures of *C. pyogenes, P. indolicus* and *Str. dysgalactiae* and examined the length of time that these bacteria could be recovered from the fly. *C. pyogenes* persisted in the fly for at least 16 days, *Str. dysgalactiae* for between 8 and 16 days, but they were unsuccessful in infecting flies with *P. indolicus*.

In conclusion, of the 40 to 50 diptera visiting cattle only a handfull have, up to now, been demonstrated to carry the pathogens commonly identified in summer mastitis secretions. Moreover, four species — *S. calcitrans, Haematobia irritans, H. meteorica* and *M. autumnalis* are asynchronous in their population dynamics with the disease incidence curve and are thus unlikely to function as vectors. On these grounds the sole remaining potential vectors are *H. irritans*, and some unidentified *Simulium* spp. and *Culicoides* spp. Summer mastitis pathogens are found at much higher frequencies in *Hydrotaea* than in the latter two species groups. Moreover, both Simuliidae and Ceratopogonidae are relatively more abundant than *H. irritans* in low incidence areas than high incidence areas in Denmark (Nielsen *et al.*, 1985a; see also Fig. 1, Overgaard Nielsen *et al.*, this section). This tends to support the case for the involvement of *H. irritans* in the transmission of summer mastitis but more quantitative and taxonomic data are needed regarding the above mentioned biting flies.

6. Artificial transmission experiments

Although the material reviewed above in part 5 indicates clearly that summer mastitis pathogens can be recovered from *H. irritans* for considerable periods after being imbibed, this does not necessarily imply that the fly can function as a vector and transmit the bacteria. This can only be demonstrated by carrying out artificial or actual transmission experiments. Artificial experiments were carried out using *H. irritans* as a vector by Thomas and Hillerton in 1984 (unpublished results) in which sterile flies were offered a bacterially "spiced meal" and allowed to feed on a sterile substrate after different time intervals. Successful transmission of *C. pyogenes* was obtained for at least two days. Attempts to do this with *P. indolicus* failed. Madsen and Sorensen (1985) were successful in obtaining artificial transmission of both *C. pyogenes* and *P. indolicus* for periods up to 7 days, and both Hillerton (pers. comm.) and Thomas *et al.* (see this section) later achieved transmission of both above mentioned bacteria. All these results show clearly that, under controlled conditions at least, *Hydrotaea irritans* is indeed capable of acting as a vector for summer mastitis pathogens.

7. Actual transmission experiments

The ultimate evidence involving *H. irritans* in summer mastitis epidemics is a successful actual transmission experiment. Successful attempts have been reported on three occasions, twice by Stuart and Parish (1955, 1956) and later by Tarry *et al.* (1978). On all three attempts the success ratio was high. Unfortunately, the details given in the reports are sparce and numerous attempts to replicate the experiments have failed in England, Denmark and The Netherlands.

CONCLUSION

As far as the endogenous hypothesis is concerned, although latent, subclinical infections have been shown to be present in healthy animals, there appears to be insufficient evidence extantly available to draw any firm conclusions regarding its validity. In other words, the hypothesis remains to be tested and more information is required, particularly regarding the distribution of endogenous infections in relation to local summer mastitis and non-summer mastitis areas, the mechanism by which the pathogens are dispersed through the population and the nature of the season specific triggering mechanism. It is only then that any decision can be made as to its validity and as to whether the hypothesis is indeed totally mutually exclusive to one involving vector transmission by cattle flies, and specifically by *H. irritans*. Although the evidence on which the latter is based is largely correlative, its very bulk completely reduces the possibility that it is simply coincidental. Given the information currently available one cannot help but to conclude that summer mastitis is a vector transmitted disease and that it is extremely probable that *Hydrotaea irritans* is the species involved, at least in the palaeoarctic region.

VECTOR BIOLOGY OF FLIES ON GRAZING CATTLE IN GERMANY

A. Liebisch

Institute of Parasitology,
Department of Veterinary Entomology,
Veterinary School Hannover,
Bunteweg 17, D – 3000 Hannover, F.R.G.

ABSTRACT

Flies (Muscidae) and tabanids (Tabanidae) associated with grazing cattle were studied in North Germany over a period of 5 years (1982–1986). Of the 19 species of flies and 20 species of tabanids infesting cattle during the pasturing season the species *Haematobia irritans* and *H. stimulans* (60-80%), *Hydrotaea irritans* and *H. albipuncta* (10-50%) and *Musca autumnalis* (30%) were found to be most abundant. *Haematopota pluvialis* and *H. italica* were the most abundant tabanid species. The seasonal activity of the more important Diptera and other biological features were studied. *Corynebacterium pyogenes* could be isolated from the viscera of 323 singly identified, dissected and examined flies belonging to the species *Hydrotaea irritans* (3.4%), *Musca autumnalis* (1.5%) and *H. meridionalis* (0.3%).

INTRODUCTION

There is only very little basic information available on the fauna of symbovine flies in Germany, the abundance of the fly species, their seasonal activity and vector relationship. When we started our study into flies on grazing cattle in Germany (Elger and Liebisch, 1982; Liebisch and Elger, 1983) we relied on earlier work done in Denmark (Hammer, 1941), England (Kirkwood and Tarry, 1973) and Scotland (Titchener et al., 1981). Concerning flies in Germany, we found the fundamental taxonomic works of Lindner (1949), Hennig (1964), and some brief studies on symbovine Diptera in the eastern (Ziegler, 1970) and in the southern part of the country (Mair, 1980; Mayer, 1981) useful. The present paper briefly summarizes an important part of the studies done during the years 1981 – 1986. Other parts of the work are published in the theses of Michael (1983) and Elger (1985) as well as in some other papers of the same school.

MATERIALS AND METHODS

Most of the studies were conducted in an enclosed area to the north-west of Hannover, Germany. The area is exclusively used as grassland for pasturing cattle. It is about 30 km in diameter, and most parts belong to a landscape preservation area. In ecological terms the area consists of moor and woodland, part of it drained. The meadows are marshy and traversed by ditches, with smaller areas of woodland and moorland between. Ticks *(Ixodes ricinus)*, flies and tabanids abound. Babesiosis *(B. divergens)* and summer mastitis in cattle are endemic.

In the centre of the area, on a pasture owned by our institute, a special herd of Friesian cattle is kept for the purpose of catching Diptera associated with the cattle. These animals had become accustomed to the presence of research workers over a period of years, and do not resist the catching procedures. A number of studies on the diptera fauna in cattle, seasonal and daily activities, host preferences, infestation sites, resting places on the hosts, breeding sites and disease relationships were carried out in this way.

For purpose of the present studies fly counts were performed weekly. The count was taken on standing animals only, on one side and on the head. For easy field diagnosis the following species could be distinguished on the animal at a distance of 2 m or less: *Haematobia irritans, H. stimulans, Musca autumnalis, Hydrotaea* spec., *Morellia* spec., *Haematopota* spec., *Hybomitra* spec., *Heptatoma* spec. and *Chrysops* spec. Species of Diptera were identified under the microscope using the taxonomic works of Hucket (1954), Hennig (1964), Zumpt (1973), Moucha and Chvála (1968), Chvála *et al.* (1972) and Peus (1980). Fly counts of the 5 years were pooled, and the arithmetical mean is presented in the diagrams.

No fly counts were made on rainy days. It was postponed until the next fine day. The weather data, temperature, humidity and rainfall were continuously measured in the grazing area. Light intensity and wind velocity were measured and cloud situation was assessed during the time of count.

RESULTS

Here are reported only the results concerning the most abundant species of flies and tabanids on cattle related to the transmission of diseases. More detailed faunistic and biological information is presented by Elger (1985).

During our faunistic studies in North Germany on grazing cattle we found 5 genera of flies (Muscidae) including 19 species which are closely related and associated with cattle (Table 1).

TABLE 1.   **Flies (Muscidae) associated with cattle in Germany**

Haematobia irritans L.,	*Hydrotaea palaestrica* Meigen
Haematobia stimulans Meigen,	*Hydrotaea pellucens* Portschinsky
Hydrotaea albipuncta Zetterstedt,	*Hydrotaea occulta* Meigen
Hydrotaea armipes Fallén,	*Hydrotaea tuberculata* Rondani
Hydrotaea bimaculata Meigen,	*Morellia hortorum* Fallén
Hydrotaea dentipes Fabricius,	*Morellia podagrica* Loew
Hydrotaea irritans Fallén,	*Morellia simplex* Loew
Hydrotaea meridionalis Portschinsky,	*Musca autumnalis* Degeer
Hydrotaea meteorica L.,	*Stomoxys calcitrans* L.
Hydrotaea militaris Meigen,	

Most prevalent are the 2 species of biting flies *Haematobia irritans* (horn fly) and *H. stimulans*, which together contribute as much as 60% (spring, summer) to 80% (late summer, autumn) to the total fly population. *H. irritans* is by far the most prevalent species, with dense populations throughout the year.

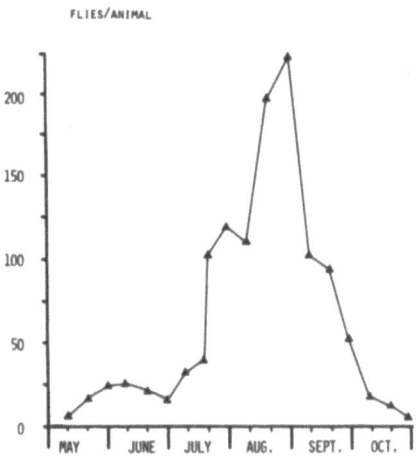

Fig. 1. Seasonal fluctuation of *Haematobia irritans*.

Peak activities are seen from mid- July until mid- September with the culmination point at the end of August (Fig. 1). The species is most closely linked with the cattle host. The imagines live on it, and leave only to lay eggs. Their nutrient medium is cattle blood, and the cattle faeces neccessarily serve as nutrient medium and habitat for the larvae.

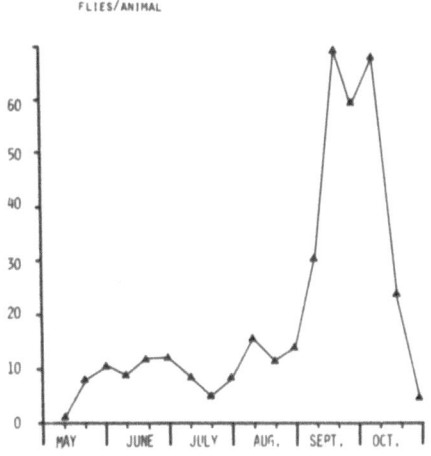

Fig. 2. Seasonal fluctuation of *Haematobia stimulans*.

The bigger species of biting fly, *Haematobia stimulans*, continues to increase in number during spring and summer into the autumn without attacking in the same large numbers as horn flies. It is also closely linked with the cattle host, sucking blood from it, and present on the host at least during the day time. Cattle faeces serve as the nutrient medium for the larvae, and constitute their habitat.

The face fly, *Musca autumnalis* is at its peak in July-August (Fig. 3), on account of the brief development period of the pre-imaginal stages (only 2 weeks) at a season in which the highest temperatures are recorded. *Musca autumnalis* is very evident on the head, and concentrates on the area around the eyes. Flies on the eyes were present throughout almost the entire study period, and their temperature-dependence was particularly evident. During July and August this species accounts for at least 30% of all flies on cattle.

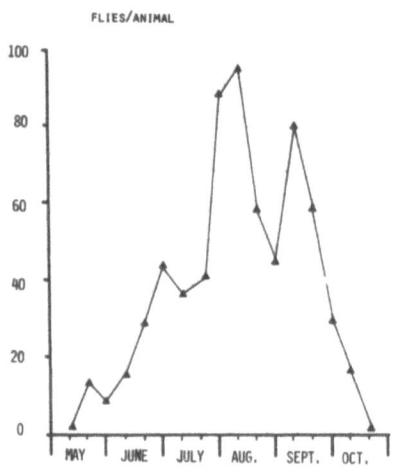

Fig. 3. Seasonal fluctuation of *Musca autumnalis*.

Flies of the genus *Hydrotaea* were represented by 12 species. However the 2 species *Hydrotaea irritans* and *H. albipuncta* together account for about 90% of all flies of this genus. They represent between 10 and 15% of all flies infesting the cattle. There is a marked difference in the seasonal activity of the 2 species. *H. irritans* is an unimodal species, building up to peak activity during July and August (Fig. 4). *H. albipuncta* shows a bimodal seasonal dynamic, making a first peak in early June and a second peak in mid-September (Fig. 5). The latter shows a low abundance in July/August, just during the peak abundance of *H. irritans*. Because of the same food site preference of the 2 species, feeding competition may be an explanation for the different activity patterns.

Flies of the genus *Morellia* were represented by 3 species. Alltogether these flies were less abundant, making up less than 20% of all fly counts on cattle.

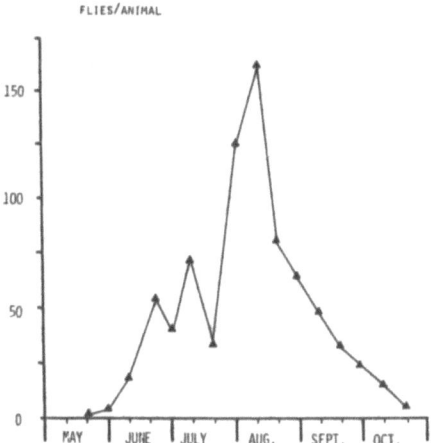

Fig. 4. Seasonal fluctuation of *Hydrotaea irritans*.

Of the 20 species of tabanids occurring in the area (Elger, 1985: Table 2) only the 2 small *Heamatopota* species, *H. italica* and *H. pluvialis*, are present in any numbers, and these species are mainly responsible for the plague of tabanids (Fig. 6). The maximum incidence of *Haematopota* occurred in the fine weather of July and August. A few varieties of *Hybomitra* and *Haeptatoma* appeared from the end of May and a few *Chrysops* from the end of June, though neither these nor *Tabanus* reached any significant proportions.

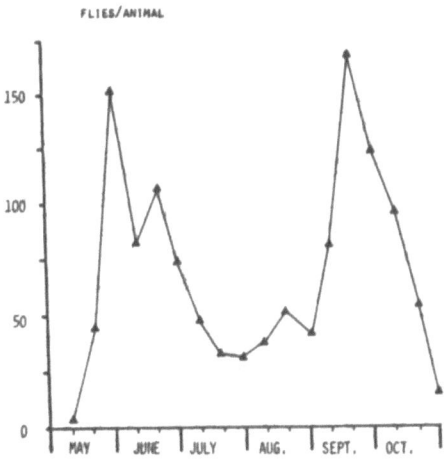

Fig. 5. Seasonal fluctuation of *Hydrotaea albipuncta*.

In spite of the low abundance of the bigger tabanids, *Hybomitra bimaculata*, the most prevalent species of the bigger tabanids, was very often recognized feeding on the teats of heifers and cows. The extravasated blood was greedily licked by *Hydrotaea irritans, Hydrotaea albipuncta* and *Musca autumnalis*. Sometimes more than 20 fresh and older bloody dots, the results of tabanid bites, could be seen on one single teat.

TABLE 2.   **Horse flies (Tabanidae) on cattle in Germany**

Chrysops caecutiens L.,	*Hybomitra ciureai* Seguy
Chrysops pictus Meigen,	*Hybomitra distiguenda* Verral
Chrysops relictus Meigen,	*Hybomitra lundbecki* Lyneborg
Heptatoma pellucens Fabricius,	*Hybomitra micans* Meigen
Haematopota crassicornis Wahlenberg,	*Hybomitra montana* Meigen
Haematopota italica Meigen,	*Tabanus bromius* L.
Haematopota pluvialis L.,	*Tabanus bovinus* L.
Haematopota subcylindrica Pandellé	*Tabanus glaucopis* Meigen
Hybomitra arpadi Szilady,	*Tabanus maculicornis* Zetterstedt
Hybomitra bimaculata Macquart	*Tabanus sudeticus* Zeller

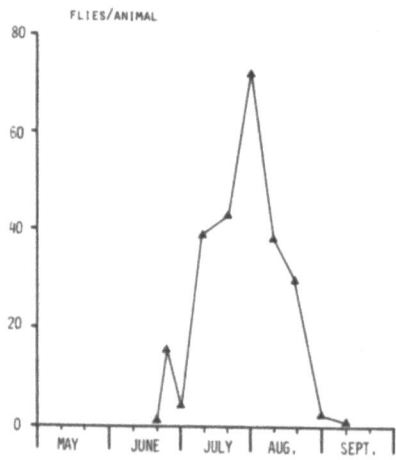

Fig. 6. Seasonal fluctuation of *Haematopota* spec. (mainly *Haematopota italica* and *Haematopota pluvialis*).

In further studies in the same Hannover area in cooperation with the Department of Udder Diseases of the Veterinary School Hannover (Head: Prof. Dr. U. Weigt), flies of the genus *Hydrotaea* and *Musca autumnalis* were examined for *C. pyogenes* (Michael, 1983). Altogether 323 flies were caught, identified and separately dissected. Flies caught on the udders belonged mainly to the species *H. irritans*. After complete dissection and examination, *C. pyogenes* was isolated from the viscera of 11 *H. irritans* (3.4%), 1 *H. meridionalis* (0.3%) and 5 *Musca autumnalis* (1.5%). Altogether 17 flies (5.3%) proved to be infected. These findings demonstrate, that at least under German conditions, the mentioned fly species must be considered as potential vectors of *C. pyogenes*.

THE FLY FAUNA OF HEIFERS AND THE TRANSMISSION OF SUMMER MASTITIS IN DENMARK

B. Overgaard Nielsen*, S.A. Nielsen**, J. Jespersen***

*Institute of Zoology and Zoophysiology,
Universitetsparken, DK–8000 Aarhus C, Denmark.
** Institute I, Roskilde University Center,
Roskilde, Denmark.
*** Danish Pest Infestation Laboratory,
Lyngby, Denmark.

ABSTRACT

A total of 44 species of Diptera was recorded from pasturing heifers in Denmark. The sheep head fly *(Hydrotaea irritans)*, the biting flies *Haematobosca stimulans* and *Lyperosia irritans*, two species of biting midges (Ceratopogonidea) and a black fly species (Simuliidae) were predominant. The species composition of the fly fauna and the density of the species observed varied during the day and regionally. A relation between the abundance of *Hydrotaea irritans* and the incidence of summer mastitis in pastures was observed. The seasonal activity and the distribution of insects over the bodies of heifers were studied. Since *Hydrotaea irritans* is abundant on the udder at the correct time of the year, this fly is most likely to be involved in the transmission of the disease. An interaction between biting and non-biting, udder-visiting flies is suggested.

INTRODUCTION

In 1979, a multidisciplinary research project on summer mastitis was initiated by the Danish Agricultural and Veterinary Research Council which included entomological investigations on the fly fauna of pasturing heifers. The purpose of the latter part of the project was to identify species of Diptera, which might be involved in the transmission of the disease. It was assumed that a temporal and regional coincidence between the incidence of summer mastitis and the abundance and acitvity of the insects involved occurred and only insect species regularly visiting the udder of heifers were suspected.

This paper reports on the fauna of Diptera recorded from heifers pasturing in different types of grassland, the daily and seasonal variation in abundance and activity of the flies observed and the distribution of the species over the bodies of the heifers. Only a few main results are presented; details will be published in future papers (in preparation).

METHODS

The entomological investigations were primarily carried out in the pastures of Store Vildmose, Northern Jutland, being the main research site of the Danish summer mastitis project 1979-1982. In Store Vildmose (area about 775 ha) about 3000 heifers are pastured annually. In the summer of 1979 and 1980 sampling was also done in 17 pastures of different environmental conditions situated in various parts of Jutland. Nearly all heifers belonged to the Black and White Dairy cattle race (SDM).

The insects were collected by: 1) Standardized sweeping just above the head and the back and along the belly of heifers, respectively, and by: 2) Vacuum cleaning of head, back, flanks, belly, udder and front legs separately for 3 minutes. In order to collect as many insect species — above all species of biting midges — as possible, all sampling was carried out on tethered heifers. Since the avoidance reactions of the heifers were hampered by this procedure, the activity and density of some fly species on untethered heifers were recorded in a large number of pastures by means of binoculars.

RESULTS

The fauna of Diptera visiting pasturing heifers

More than 50.000 Diptera representing 44 species were recorded from heifers, viz. 18 species of biting midges (Ceratopogonidae), 5 species of black flies (Simuliidae), 6 species of horse flies (Tabanidae) and 15 species of Muscidae. The sheep head fly (*Hydrotaea irritans* Fall.), black flies of the *Simulium ornatum*-species complex, the biting midges *Culicoides scoticus* Downes & Kettle and *C. obsoletus* Mg. and the biting flies *Haematobosca stimulans* (Mg.) and *Lyperosia irritans* L. contributed more than 85% of all Diptera recorded.

Diurnal and regional variation in the fly fauna

The species composition of the dipterous fauna of heifers changed in the course of the day and between the pastures (Fig. 1).

Nearly all species of biting midges were mainly recorded on the heifers at sunset and sunrise, the black flies were chiefly active on the cattle in late afternoon and early in the evening and the biting flies *Lyperosia irritans* and *Haematobosca stimulans* as well as the sheep head fly were recorded from early morning to late evening.

In some of the pastures biting midges only contributed < 10%, in others 60-75% of the crepuscular fauna (Fig. 1). In the majority of the pastures the activity of black flies was negligible, but in a few sites these insects made up > 65% of the fly fauna (Fig. 1). The relative abundance of *Lyperosia irritans* and *Hydrotaea irritans* varied regionally from about 1% to nearly 80% of the total fauna recorded (Fig. 1).

For each predominant taxon of Diptera the mean number of individuals per sample per site was calculated. The sum of the mean numbers expressed the "insect burden" of heifers pasturing under different environmental conditions. The "insect burden" varied considerably. For instance in two of the sites, *e.g.* in Store Vildmose, the density of *Hydrotaea irritans* was remarkably high, whereas an extremely low density was recorded in some coastal grassland areas, *e.g.* Vaern Enge (Nielsen *et al.*, 1985a).

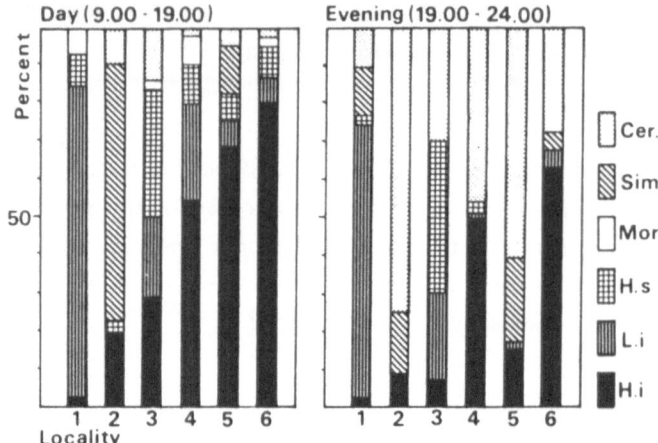

Fig. 1. The relative abundance of taxa of Diptera in 6 Danish grassland sites during the day and in the evening. H.i. = *Hydrotaea irritans*, L.i. = *Lyperosia irritans*, H.s. = *Haematobosca stimulans*, Mor. = *Morellia* spp., Sim. = Simuliidae, Cer. = Ceratopogonidae. Locality I = Vaern Enge, Locality 6 = Store Vildmose.

The seasonal activity of flies

All predominant species of biting midges and black flies, the biting flies *Haematobosca stimulans* and *Lyperosia irritans* and the sheep head fly were observed on heifers from May to October, however, the seasonal maximum in population density of the species differed. Biting midges and black flies were most abundant in July-August and May-June, respectively. In *H. stimulans* apparently two seasonal maxima occurred, *viz.* in May-June and September, the numbers being maximal in the latter period. The number of *L. irritans* and *H. irritans* increased from June to a peak in July-August.

Distribution of Diptera over the bodies of heifers

The distribution of 16 abundant species of Diptera over the bodies of heifers was analyzed. The density of each species per square unit of skin surface was calculated and the difference in density recorded between body parts was tested (multiple range, multiple F-test) (Table 1). *Culicoides scoticus* was primarily recorded on the head and back, *Culicoides obsoletus*, *C. punctatus* and the *Simulium ornatum*-species complex on the belly and the udder. The densities of male and female *Lyperosia irritans* were significantly higher on the flanks and the back and on the flanks only, respectively, than on all other parts of the heifer's body. *Haematobosca stimulans* (♂♂ and ♀♀) was most abundant on the legs.

Generally, the density of *Hydrotaea irritans* was significantly higher on the lower body parts (legs, belly and udder), than on the upper ones (head, back and flanks), however, the distribution pattern of the sheep head fly varied between pastures. In some sites the density of *Hydrotaea irritans* was significantly higher on the head than on the back and flanks and in Store Vildmose not significantly different from the densities observed on the lower body parts (Table 1). The distribution patterns of *Lyperosia irritans* and *Hydrotaea irritans* recorded on tethered and untethered heifers were practically the same (Table 1).

TABLE 1.　Distribution of species of Diptera over the bodies of tethered and untethered heifers; with three exceptions data from all sites are pooled: F: Data from Funder, Central Jutland, V: Data from Store Vildmose. *Abundance significantly higher than in all other parts of the heifer's body ($p < 0.05$) (for details, see Nielsen *et al.*, 1985b).

	N	head	back	% flanks	belly	udder	legs
A. Tethered							
C. obsoletus	937	9.0	4.2	2.1	*60.5	11.1	13.2
C. punctatus	237	1.8	1.6	0.7	*49.3	*36.6	10.0
(F) C. scoticus	489	*32.5	*39.8	8.3	7.8	5.4	6.2
S. ornatum	9730	1.4	0.1	0.3	*56.3	*38.5	3.5
H. stimulans (♀♀)	333	0.0	6.1	27.0	3.2	0.0	*63.7
L. irritans (♀♀)	202	0.0	22.4	*62.6	11.4	2.5	1.1
(V) H. irritans	9623	*14.8	3.5	3.9	*31.6	*27.0	*19.3
(F) H. irritans	2436	8.4	0.7	2.7	*43.7	*22.7	*21.8
B. Untethered							
L. irritans	1665	0.0	34.6	49.6	14.8	0.1	0.9
H. irritans	1892	25.2	6.7	14.9	26.5	16.5	10.2

The niche breadth (Colwell and Futuyma, 1971) of the fly species showed that *e.g. Haematobosca stimulans, Lyperosia irritans* and *Simulium ornatum* were aggregated on a few body parts, whereas *Hydrotaea irritans* was more uniformly distributed over the bodies of the heifers, especially in Store Vildmose. A high niche overlap (Colwell and Futuyma, *op. cit.*) was observed between *e.g. Hydrotaea irritans, Culicoides obsoletus, C. punctatus, Simulium ornatum* and mosquitoes (Culicidae), especially on the udder. However, the pattern of niche overlap observed varied regionally.

DISCUSSION

The species composition of the fly fauna of heifers varied between pastures. Above all, the relative abundance and density of the sheep head fly varied regionally. Since this fly is under suspicion of being involved in the transmission of summer mastitis, a relation between the spatial variation in the incidence of the disease and in the density of the sheep head fly on heifers is crucial. For instance, in Vaern Enge, where the abundance of *H. irritans* is extremely low the incidence of summer mastitis is nil. In Store Vildmose, however, the sheep head fly is abundant and summer mastitis is a recurrent problem (Madsen *et al.*, 1986). These observations suggest that some relation between the abundance of *Hydrotaea irritans* and the incidence of summer mastitis in a site may exist.

Generally, the peak incidence of summer mastitis is in late July-early August; consequently, insect species active on heifers during this time of the summer are those most likely to be involved in the transmission of the disease. *Lyperosia irritans, Hydrotaea irritans* and all predominant species of biting midges are abundant at the correct time. Apart from a mutual displacement of 10 days, the seasonal feeding activity of the sheep head flies on heifers and the temporal prevalence of summer mastitis changed alike (Madsen, *et al.*, 1986).

Four species of Diptera occurred regularly on the teats of heifers, *viz.* 2 species of biting midges, a black fly and the sheep head fly. Since the pathogens responsible for summer mastitis can be carried by the latter species, but apparently only on rare occasions by biting flies (Bahr, 1952; Sorensen, 1974; Hillerton *et al.*, 1983; Madsen, 1985) the sheep head fly is further incriminated. However, the overlap of body site occupied by biting and non-biting flies may be an important factor in the transmission of summer mastitis, at least in some pastures, the sheep head fly being attracted by primary damage caused by biting flies.

Based on the entomological investigations carried out, the circumstantial evidence for the involvement of *Hydrotaea irritans* in the transmission of summer mastitis is strong.

HEIFER MASTITIS IN SWEDEN DURING A THREE YEAR PERIOD (1982–1985): ENTOMOLOGICAL ASPECTS

J. Chirico*, P. Jonsson*,**, S–O. Olsson***, O. Holmberg*,**** and H. Funke***

*National Veterinary Institute, S–750 07 Uppsala, Sweden.
**Present address: EWOS AB, Box 618, S–151–27 Södertälje, Sweden.
***Swedish Association for Livestock Breeding and Production,
Animal Health Department, Eskilstuna, Sweden.
****Swedish University of Agricultural Sciences, Dept. of Veterinary Microbiology,
Section of Clinical Microbiology, Uppsala, Sweden.

ABSTRACT

Within the Swedish heifer mastitis project a fly survey of 48 herds distributed in 8 different geographical areas (counties) was carried out during 1983-1985. This paper is a preliminary report on the fly distribution on the udders of grazing heifers in the 8 areas investigated during 1983. The fly *Hydrotaea irritans* (Fall.) (Diptera: Muscidae), which is considered a potential transmitter of summer mastitis related bacteria, was recovered from all of the areas that were sampled. *H. irritans* was the most frequent fly species in samples from 6 out of the 8 areas investigated.

INTRODUCTION

The fly *H. irritans* (Fall.) (Diptera: Muscidae) is considered a potential mechanical transmitter of bacteria related to summer mastitis secretions (Sorensen, 1974; Wright and Titchener, 1977; Bramley *et al.*, 1985; Hillerton and Bramley, 1985; Madsen, 1985; Madsen *et al.*, 1986). One of the Danish studies points out a correlation between the prevalance periods for *H. irritans* and summer mastitis pathogens: (Madsen *et al.*, 1986). The biology of *H. irritans* and its distribution on grazing heifers also suggest that it has possible importance as a potential transmitter of the above mentioned pathogens (Overgaard-Nielsen *et al.*, 1971, 1972). Accordingly, a fly survey was included in the Swedish heifer mastitis project during 1983-1985 (Olsson *et al.*, 1986). This fly survey was the first investigation of its kind conducted on a national basis, and would contribute essential data concerning the distribution of fly species around the udders of pastured heifers. As Sweden has a wide range of climatic and geographical conditions, it was possible to investigate whether this fly fauna differs in distribution and abundance in different parts of the country.

This preliminary report concentrates on the distribution of flies within the family of Muscidae in the areas investigated in 1983.

MATERIALS AND METHODS

The present investigation included a total of 48 herds distributed equally in 8 different counties situated between approximately 55° — 63° lat. and 12° — 18° long. (Fig. 1). The sampled herds represented previous occurrence of mastitis, and not (or in very low frequency) mastitis affected herds in equal proportions (3+3).

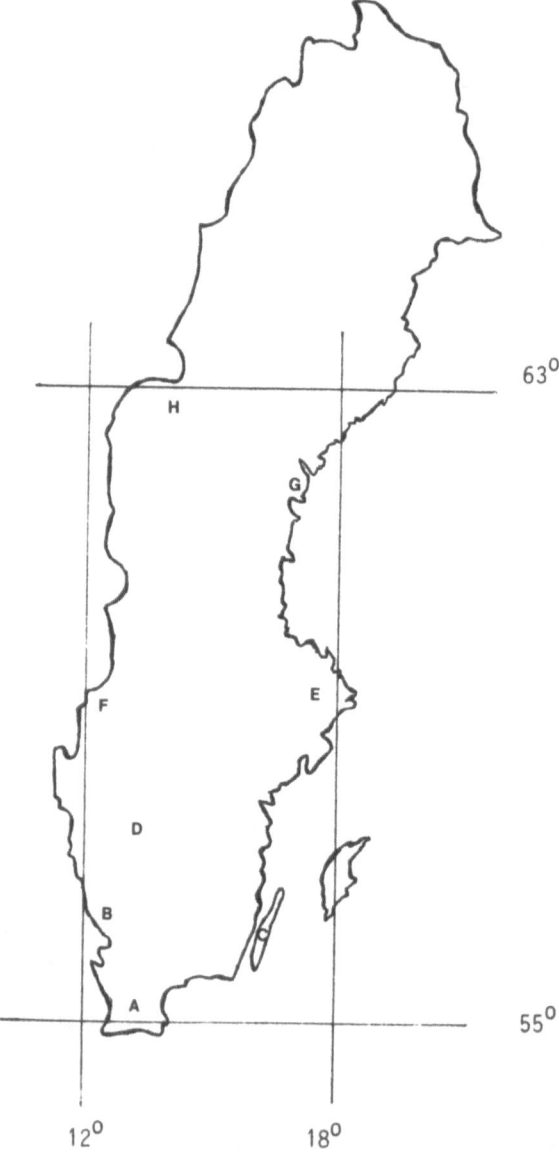

Fig. 1. A. Hörby, B. Falkenberg, C. Öland, D. Falköping, E. Uppsala, F. Arvika/Åarjäng, G. Nyland, H. Mansasen/Berg.

Fly samples around heifer udders were taken using hand nets for half an hour every fortnight between mid-June and mid-September. Sampled flies were kept in 70% alcohol for subsequent identification.

RESULTS

TABLE 1. **The total prevalence of Muscidae with special reference to** *H. irritans,* *H. albipuncta, Ha. irritans* **and** *Ha. stimulans.*

Area	Fly sp.	Nos.	%	Area	Fly sp.	Nos.	%
A*	H. irr.	978	84.02	B*	H. irr.	1394	74.07
	H. alb.	23	1.98		H. alb.	42	2.23
	Ha. irr.	21	1.80		Ha. irr.	27	1.44
	Ha. stim.	25	2.15		Ha. stim.	45	2.39
	Rest.	117	10.05		Rest.	374	19.87
	Tot.	1164			Tot.	1882	
C*	H. irr.	203	2.16	D*	H. irr.	2625	76.62
	H. alb.	8	0.09		H. alb.	89	2.60
	Ha. irr.	8901	94.69		Ha. irr.	3	0.09
	Ha. stim.	97	1.03		Ha. stim.	17	0.49
	Rest.	191	2.03		Rest.	690	20.20
	Tot.	9400			Tot.	3426	
E*	H. irr.	2005	49.74	F*	H. irr.	336	35.04
	H. alb.	158	3.92		H. alb.	53	5.53
	Ha. irr.	33	0.82		Ha. irr.	—	—
	Ha. stim.	749	18.58		Ha. stim.	22	2.29
	Rest.	1086	26.94		Rest.	548	57.14
	Tot.	4031			Tot.	959	
G*	H. irr.	505	46.76	H*	H. irr.	906	51.98
	H. alb.	31	2.87		H. alb.	126	7.23
	Ha. irr.	—	—		Ha. irr.	—	—
	Ha. stim.	317	29.30		Ha. stim.	317	18.19
	Rest.	227	21.00		Rest.	394	22.60
	Tot.	1080			Tot.	1743	

*= Areas see Fig. 1.

A total of 23, 685 flies of the family Muscidae were collected. The fly species found during the investigation were *Haematobia irritans* (L.), *Haematobosca (Haematobia) stimulans*

(Meig.), *Hydrotaea albipuncta* (Zett.), *H. armipes* (Fall.), *H. borussica* (Stein.), *H. cinerea* (RD), *H. irritans* (Fall.), *H. meridionalis* (Portsch.), *H. meteorica* (L.), *H. militaris* (Meig.), *H. pandellei* (Stein.), *H. pellucens* (Portsch.), *H. pilitibia* (Stein.), *H. tuberculata* (Rond.), *H. velutina* (RD), *Morellia hortorum* (Fall.), *M. simplex* (Loew.) *Musca autumnalis* (DeG.), *M. domestica* (L.), *Pogonomyia (Trichopticoides) decolor* (Fall.), and *Stomoxys calcitrans* (L.).

As there are certain references to some fly species when discussing the summer mastitis complex, Table 1 shows the prevalence of *H. irritans, H. albipuncta, Ha. irritans*, and *Ha. stimulans*.

These were the four most common fly species in all of the areas investigated except area F, where *M. autumnalis* was the most frequent species. *H. irritans* was the most abundant Muscidae in all of the areas except areas C and F.

DISCUSSION

The fly *H. irritans* is present in all investigated areas. Accordingly it is obvious that Sweden harbours this potential transmitter of summer mastitis pathogens. The appearance, prevalence, and bacteriological constitution of heifer mastitis in Sweden differs from that in Denmark and W. Germany (Olsson *et al.*, 1986; Jonsson *et al.*, 1986; Madsen, 1985; Tolle *et al.*, 1983). This preliminary study suggests, however, that the fly fauna in Sweden does not differ from that in other countries where fly surveys of this kind have been carried out.

Within the survey carried out during the past three years, additional data have been collected that may help explain the importance of certain environmental factors in the distribution and abundance of the fly species present, such as: 1. temperature and wind speed; 2. topographical character of the pastures; 3. type of vegetation present; 4. presence of water, *e.g.* lakes and streams; 5. type of drinking facilities; 6. number of heifers present; 7. composition of the race within each herd. To correlate the above mentioned entomological information with the incidence of summer mastitis within the herds studied, data concerning the appearance and determination of bacteria present have been recorded in all cases of mastitis. All these parameters are currently being statistically analysed by the "Statistic Analysis System" (SAS) and are being subjected to an analysis of variance (the GLM procedure). Presumably this computer analysis will clarify the relationship between the above environmental parameters and the outbreak of summer mastitis.

ACKNOWLEDGEMENTS

The Farmers Research Council for Information and Development financially supported this work.

CHROMOSOME AND ENZYME VARIATION OF *HYDROTAEA IRRITANS* (FALLEN) (DIPTERA: MUSCIDAE)

V. Loeschke*, B. Overgaard Nielsen**, B. Christensen***,

V. Simonsen*, S.A. Nielsen**** and D. Anderson*

*Institute of Ecology and Genetics, University of Aarhus,
Ny Munkegade, DK—8000 Aarhus C, Denmark.
**Institute of Zoology and Zoophysiology, University of Aarhus,
Aarhus, Denmark.
***Institute of Population Biology, University of Copenhagen,
Denmark.
****Institute of Biological Chemistry, Roskilde University,
Roskilde, Denmark.

ABSTRACT

The analysis of metaphases from the brain of third instar larvae from flies caught in the Netherlands revealed numbers of chromosomes ranging from 12 to 15. Of these, five pairs of large metacentric and submetacentric chromosomes were common to all individuals, so the number of supernumerous chromosomes varied from 2 to 5. In an ongoing study of variation in chromosome number of flies caught in Denmark, we found two common types each with 12 and one rare type with 11 chromosomes in forest flies. In the majority of flies from nearby pastures, we counted 13 or 14 chromosomes, but larvae with 12 or 11 chromosomes were also found.

Variation in isozyme frequencies was investigated by electrophoresis in populations from several locations in Jutland (Denmark). Each locality was represented by a sample from a forest area and a nearby pasture. The data revealed a peculiar banding pattern at four enzyme loci. The occurrence of certain presumed heteroxygous bands at one of these loci was linked to the occurrence of certain other presumed heterozygous bands at the other three loci. Despite rather high frequencies of such "heterotypes", at least in some samples, one of the corresponding homozygote types was never observed. The banding pattern at another polymorphic locus was independent of the occurrence of "heterotypes".

Possible hypotheses to explain the observed pattern of variation are discussed.

INTRODUCTION

The genetic analysis of insect pest populations can reveal information on population structure and on the mode of reproduction that may be of importance in pest control. Here we report on a study on chromosome and enzyme variation in populations of *Hydrotaea irritans* from Denmark and the Netherlands.

CHROMOSOMAL VARIATION

Larvae from flies swept on one day in August, 1985 in the Staphorst area in the Netherlands (provided by Dr. G. Thomas, Lelystad, The Netherlands) and during summer 1986 in the Lovenholm forest and on nearby pastures in Eastern Jutland, Denmark, were used for the analysis of chromosomes. Standard procedures were applied for slide preparations and only preparations that contained at least 10 metaphases, which allowed unambiguous counting of chromosome number, were used. In these preparations, number and shape of chromosomes were consistent within slides.

Flies from the Netherlands

Among 9 larvae the number of chromosomes varied between 12 and 15 (Fig. 1). The type with 13 chromosomes was most common and occurred in five of the nine preparations. Five pairs of large metacentric and submetacentric chromosomes were common to all preparations. The remaining chromosomes were smaller and acrocentric and did not necessarily occur in pairs (for more details see Loeschke and Christensen, 1986). The variation in chromosome number resembles that of B-chromosomes known from flowering plants and animals (for review see Jones and Rees, 1982). Sex chromosomes were not identified in this investigation.

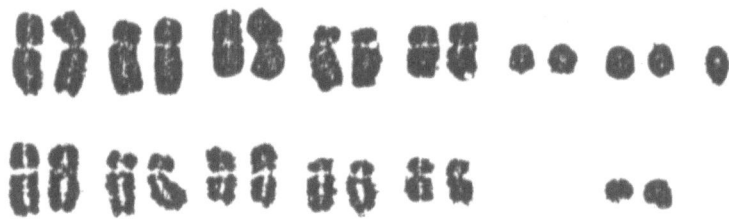

Fig. 1. Karyograms of two of the observed types exhibiting 12 and 15 chromosomes.

Flies from Denmark

The analysis of chromosomes of the Danish flies has not yet been finished. In the first preparations of larvae of 22 flies caught in Lovenholm forest we found that these have 11 or 12 chromosomes of which again five pairs seem to be common to all individuals. In the 12 chromosome case the remaining two chromosomes seem to consist either of an acrocentric pair (6 individuals so far) or a single acrocentric and a submetacentric chromosome (5 individuals). The individual with 11 chromosomes had only a single acrocentric chromosome.

Flies caught around cattle in nearby pastures however, show different variation in chromosome number. Again five pairs of metacentric and submetacentric chromosomes are common in these flies, resembling those from the forest populations, and, as far as we can tell at the moment, also those of the Dutch flies. Among 13 larvae so far investigated, we found 5 with 13 and 5 with 14 chromosomes, as well as 2 with 12 and 1 with 11 chromosomes.

ENZYME VARIATION

For the analysis of enzyme variation we used flies caught at three different locations in Denmark: Southern Jutland around Abild, Western Jutland around Skaerbaek and Eastern Jutland around Lovenholm. At each of these locations we sampled in pastures around cattle and in the nearby forest. Adult flies were brought alive to the laboratory and frozen at −70°C. Before running gels the flies were identified according to species and sex. Among about 20 enzymes studied, five were highly polymorphic and easy to score. These were: ACON (Aconitase), AMY (Amylase), FUM (Fumerase), GPI (Glucose phosphate isomerase) and PGM (Phosphoglucomutase). AMY was run on ultra thin layer focusing gels, according to Radola (1980), whereas all the other systems were run on horizontal starch gels according to routine procedures (see, *e.g.*, Frydenberg and Simonsen, 1973).

A sample from Lovenholm forest

We will focus on a sample from Lovenholm forest, caught on August 17, 1985. To point out the peculiar banding pattern revealed by electrophoresis we give the original data set for the above mentioned five enzymes (Table 1). Among the 71 flies of the sample, 37 were heterozygote for genotype 13 in ACON. Of these 37, all but one (fly No. 4) were also heterozygote in FUM for genotype 12 and in GPI for genotypes 14 or 44* (and in one case genotype 4*6). The genotype 44* in GPI shows only two of the three bands of genotype 14 and 4*6 shows the same two plus a slower band. In PGM only 31 out of the 37 flies were heterozygote for genotype 13. The remaining 6 flies were also heterozygote, but for either genotype 35 (in four cases), 34 (one case), or 23 (one case).

In two other flies we found genotypes 12 in FUM and 14 in GPI (flies No. 60 and 66) together with a heterozygote in PGM (genotype 23 or 35) and a heterozygote in ACON (genotype 24 or 34). Another fly being heterozygote 14 in GPI was unscorable in FUM and heterozygote for genotype 34 in ACON and 35 in PGM.

The data from the Lovenholm sample as well as those from other samples show a very close association of genotypes 13 in ACON, 12 in FUM, and 14 (or 44*) in GPI, and to a lesser degree with genotype 13 in PGM. We ran gels on about 1400 individuals of *H. irritans*, but not a single homozygote 11 in GPI, in ACON, or in PGM has been observed, and only 2 homozygotes 11 in FUM were recorded.

It can be excluded that the same enzyme was stained at the four loci making up the "heterotype", as there were differences in pattern and mobility between all four loci. Besides this, FUM and GPI were run on the same gel and this was also the case for PGM and ACON. When we left out the substrate for the enzymes and just added cofactors and staining chemicals no enzyme reaction was observed. We therefore conclude that the observed banding pattern is not a technical artefact but has a genetic basis.

TABLE 1.   Electromorphs at Five Enzyme Loci

FLY NO.	ACON	FUM	GPI	PGM	AMY	FLY NO.	ACON	FUM	FPI	PGM	AMY
1	13	12	14	13	22	37	33	22	44	33	55
2	33	22	44	33	44	38	13	12	14	23	44
3	13	12	14	13	11	39	33	22	44	33	14
4	13	22	44	35	13	40	13	12	14	13	22
5	33	22	44*	13	12	41	33	22	34	35	25
6	33	22	44	13	11	42	33	22	44	33	13
7	33	22	44*	35	24	43	13	12	14	13	15
8	13	12	44*	13	13	44	13	12	14	13	15
9	13	12	46*	13	33	45	13	12	14	13	13
10	13	12	44*	13	24	46	33	22	44	33	11
11	13	12	44*	34	11	47	13	12	14	35	35
12	13	12	44*	13	13	48	33	22	44	33	35
13	13	12	44*	13	55	49	33	22	44	33	33
14	13	12	44*	13	11	50	13	12	14	13	23
15	13	12	44*	13	35	51	13	12	14	13	25
16	33	22	44	33	34	52	13	12	14	13	11
17	13	12	44*	13	13	53	34	22	44	33	us
18	13	12	14	13	13	54	33	22	24	33	35
19	33	22	44	33	14	55	33	22	44	33	23
20	33	22	44*	33	13	56	34	22	44	23	35
21	33	22	44	13	22	57	13	12	14	13	15
22	13	12	14	13	13	58	13	12	14	13	44
23	13	12	14	13	13	59	13	12	14	35	33
24	13	12	44*	13	22	60	24	12	14	23	13
25	33	22	44	13	13	61	13	12	14	13	25
26	13	12	44*	13	25	62	33	22	44	35	45
27	13	12	14	13	12	63	13	12	14	13	13
28	13	12	14	13	35	64	34	us	14	13	24
29	33	22	44	33	15	65	33	22	44	23	34
30	33	22	44	13	15	66	34	12	14	35	33
31	33	22	44	33	25	67	13	12	14	13	34
32	33	22	44	33	13	68	13	12	14	13	33
33	13	12	14	35	13	69	33	22	44	33	34
34	33	22	44	13	55	70	33	22	44	33	23
35	33	22	44	35	15	71	33	22	44	33	13
36	13	12	44*	13	25						

AMY was highly variable without showing any pattern related to the genotypes at the other four loci. This remains true even when additional weaker bands not shown in the table are taken into consideration.

DISCUSSION

To explain the banding pattern revealed by gel-electrophoresis at least two phenomena have to be taken into consideration: (a) the co-occurrence of certain genotypes at several loci, and (b) the one missing homozygote.

A possible explanation for the occurrence of "heterotypes" could be close physical linkage of the loci coding for these enzymes where linkage disequilibrium is maintained by an inversion preventing recombination. The missing "homotype" has then to be explained by lethality of the monozygote for the inversion.

A modified and much less likely version of this explanation would be that the association of certain genotypes is maintained by very strong selective forces, requiring neither close physical linkage nor an inversion. Then, on the multi-locus fitness landscape, peaks are represented by the multiple heterozygote (optimum phenotype) and by one multiple homozygote. This selection scheme would impose a segregational load on the population of a magnitude which would make it unlikely for the population to survive.

Another possible explanation would be that the "heterotypes" are hybrids which are sterile or where offspring have strongly reduced fitness so that we do not find intermediate forms. This explanation, however, seems unlikely as we have not found the species that could have given rise to the observed enzyme pattern, despite running gels for all *Hydrotaea* species caught at the sampling sites and also because in some forest populations "heterotypes" made up to 50% of the population. Furthermore, in two closely related species, *Hydrotaea borusica* and *Hydrotaea albipuncta*, we also observed "heterotypes" which might indicate that "heterotypes" are phylogenetically old.

Reproduction by parthenogenesis in at least a part of the population, could also explain the occurrence of "heterotypes". As, however, one other enzyme locus, Amylase, was highly variable within "heterotypes", this explanation also seems rather unattractive.

In principle, the chromosomal variation found could account for the banding pattern revealed by electrophoresis. A chromosome that occurs only in a single copy could explain a fixed co-occurrence of certain allele types. As "heterotypes" were found among males and females, it cannot be the Y-chromosome. B-chromosomes, however, generally do not contain much DNA, so to assume four enzyme loci to be located on such a chromosome seems rather unrealistic. Still, in the face of the variation found in chromosome number, this explanation should be investigated further.

Other possible explanations include gene modifiers, post-translational modifications, or parasites. Further experiments have to be conducted to test the different hypotheses and to reveal a possible relation between the variation on the enzyme and the chromosome level. Obviously, controlled crossing experiments would be most informative in this situation. To do this on a large scale, however, requires that populations of the fly can be kept throughout the whole life cycle in the laboratory. This has not yet been done successfully. Still data on mother-offspring combinations which we are currently gathering might provide information on the segregation of "heterotypes" and on segregation of B-chromosomes.

Finally, one interesting aspect of our data should be mentioned. Electrophoretic data from the Danish flies as well as ongoing work on chromosome variation indicate a difference between forest and pasture populations, even when samples were taken only a few kilometers apart. A possible explanation of this difference could be that the "new niche" provided by cattle as a protein rich environment might have recently lead to considerable microevolutionary changes.

ACKNOWLEDGEMENT

The work has been supported by a grant from Aarhus Universitets Forskningsfond.

BACTERIAL SURVIVAL AND FEEDING PATTERN IN *HYDROTAEA IRRITANS*: TWO ESSENTIAL VARIABLES FOR A TRANSMISSION MODEL OF SUMMER MASTITIS

G. Thomas*,**, U Vecht***, J.A.J. Breeuwer**, H.J. Wisselink***
and J.N. van der Linden*

*Department of Parasitology, Central Veterinary Institute,
Postbox 65, 8200 AB Lelystad, The Netherlands.
**Department of Animal Physiology, Biological Centre, University of Groningen,
The Netherlands.
***Department of Bacteriology, Central Veterinary Institute,
Lelystad, The Netherlands.

ABSTRACT

Numerous attempts to replicate Tarry's successful transmission of summer mastitis pathogens using the sheep head fly as a vector have proved negative in England, Denmark and The Netherlands. The hypothesis is proposed that one of the reasons underlying this failure is lack of knowledge not only regarding survival of pathogens in the fly but also the feeding behaviour and hunger state of the vector. Experiments were carried out to investigate these variables. Feeding behaviour takes approximately 4 days to recover after a full meal but can be manipulated using interrupted feeding and intermeal intervals. Bacterial survival in the fly was investigated using both mixed and monocultures of summer mastitis pathogens. Successful artificial techniques were developed in which it was possible to transmit *C. pyogenes* and *P. indolicus* using artificial substrates.

INTRODUCTION

The ultimate indication involving *Hydrotaea irritans* as the vector of the causative bacteria for summer mastitis is a successful, *in vivo* transmission experiment. Manipulation of design variables can then be used to analyse the underlying transmission mechanism and thus provide valuable information for formulating a realistic epidemiological model. Successful *in vivo* transmission has been claimed on three occassions, twice by Stuart and Parish (1955, 1956) and later by Tarry *et al.* (1978). Since then, numerous attempts have been carried out in England, Denmark and The Netherlands but all of these have been unsuccessful.

It is logical that the probability of establishment of infection will be positively correlated with the bacterial load deposited in or on the quarter by the vector. Analysis of the factors that influence this is therefore essential in order to optimalize deposition. It is reasonable to assume that the probability of deposition of bacteria by an individual vector will be positively correlated with the transmission capacity of the vector and causal variables leading to its contact with the host. As female *H. irritans* visit cattle in order to obtain a protein meal, the probability of visitation and the time which they will remain in contact will be dependant on feeding motivation. As stated above, knowledge of motivational changes is, in itself, not enough to enable formulation of a realistic transmission, and eventually epidemiological, model. Transmission will also depend on the chance of bacteria being deposited. Some of the factors that are important here are: (1) how long does *H. irritans* have to feed on a bacterial substrate to cause an infection in an uninfected heifer?; (2) how long do the bacteria remain viable *and* in a transmittable site in the fly? Although literature reports state that *C. pyogenes* may be recovered from *H. irritans* females for 16 days or so (Wright and Titchener, 1977), this does not necessarily mean that the fly can transmit the bacterium for this period.

More insight is needed into these variables. This paper reports on some preliminary experiments aimed at investigating some of these.

MATERIALS AND METHODS

Flies were maintained in the laboratory in 0.25 cm^3 perspex cages on a diet of saturated sugar solution for at least two weeks before being used in an experiment.

Feeding motivation

The general experimental design used to examine changes in feeding motivation of *H. irritans* females was as follows: Flies were individually housed in 9 cm petri dishes 24 hrs prior to being offered a cattle serum meal. During this period they were deprived of sugar water and, for the last two hrs, also deprived of water. For each test, the petri dish was placed on a lighted table and 150 μl of the meal was injected into the centre of the bottom of the dish through a hole in the lid as soon as the fly reached the periphery of the dish. Intake behaviour of the fly generally consists of a rather long 1st bout followed by numerous shorter bouts interspersed with grooming, walking *etc.* (see Thomas *et al.*, 1985). The measures used in this study were the duration of the first bout and the total time the proboscis was in contact with the droplet in the three mins following the first contact.

To examine the recovery of feeding motivation for a protein meal (Exp. 1), a second serum meal was offered to the flies at intervals of 1, 2, 3 and 4 days (n = 5-10 per situation) and feeding behaviour measured again. The difference in feeding duration between 1st and 2nd meal (Δ) was determined for each fly and these data averaged for each interval class. To prevent mortality, flies were allowed to feed on saturated sugar solution 2 hrs each day between 1st and 2nd meals with the constraint that the same deprivation criteria were applied before the second meal. In order to determine how substrate influences recovery of hunger, a similar experiment was carried out using different flies. However, here the second meal consisted of defibrinated cattle blood (Exp. 2). The next experiment was directed at determining the influence of meal size on recovery of hunger (Exp. 3). The method employed was to interrupt the first meal after 5, 25 or 50 s by sucking this out of the petri dish with a syringe. As hunger might be expected to recover more quickly after the shorter meals (50 s allows a complete meal with serum) a shorter interval schedule was used and second meals offered at 6, 12, 24 and 48 hrs (n = 8 per situation).

Pathogen survival in H. irritans

To examine survival of the bacteria within the vector (Exp. 4), 128 *H. irritans* females were deprived for the same length of time as in the feeding motivation tests and then fed individually on secretion obtained from previously carried out infection experiments (see Vecht *et al.*, section 3). This secretion contained *C. pyogenes* and *P. indolicus* (2.7 x 10^9 and 2.3 x 10^9 c.f.u./ml respectively) and had been frozen at $-70°C$ and stored at $-20°C$. Half the flies were allowed to feed to repletion (> 1 min) and the remaining half underwent feeding interruption after 10 s. Eight flies were removed from each group at intervals of 0, 6, 24, 48, 96 and 168 hrs after the pathogen 'spiced' meal and examined for bacteria in batches of 4. For this, the flies were first immobilized at $-70°C$ and then washed thoroughly in 70% alcohol to remove surface contamination. Earlier experiments by Thomas and Hillerton revealed that, in general, recovery was only obtained from the interior of the fly and not the outer surface. Thereafter, they were swilled in distilled water (x2) to remove any remaining alcohol and ground in 1 ml serum bouillon in a Griffiths tube. A dilution series was made from $1-10^{-5}$ in steps of 10 using physiological saline. The liquor was plated on BHI plates and anaerobically incubated for 2 days. The data were normalized by taking the mean number of c.f.u./fly and dividing this by the number of c.f.u. in 1 ml of the original meal to give the relative number of colonies recovered per fly. The experiment was repeated using monocultures of *C. pyogenes* (6.8 x 10^7) and *P. indolicus* (3.7 x 10^8) to determine whether survival in the vector is influenced by interaction between the pathogens. An additional test was performed with a monoculture of *Streptococcus dysgalactiae* (1.2 x 10^8) (Exp. 5). These monocultures were made by culturing in BHI, centrifuging the bacteria and resuspending them in sterile, dry udder secretion. In these experiments, the flies were allowed to feed to repletion. The data were normalized in the same way as in Exp. 4.

Artificial transmission of pathogens via H. irritans

To determine whether and over what interval *H. irritans* could transmit *C. pyogenes* and *P. indolicus* the following artificial transmission experiment (Exp. 6) was carried out: two groups of 20 flies were offered a meal containing these pathogens using the same procedure and secretion as used in Experiment 4. One group was interrupted after 10 s, the other was allowed to feed to repletion in order to examine the influence of size of the pathogen meal on the pathogen load transmitted. Each group of flies was transferred into a new, sterile, 9 cm petri dish and allowed to feed on a droplet consisting of 0.2 ml of BHI for 15 mins. They were removed and kept in seperate holding cages until the next meal was due. These sterile meals were offered at 0, 1, 6, 24 and 96 hrs after feeding on the

Several tentative conclusions may be drawn from the results. Firstly, and not unexpectedly, the length of a meal has a significant influence on the time spent feeding during a subsequent meal if the interval between the two meals is short (6 hrs) (Small > Large; Medium > Large: Mann-Whitney U test, p< 0.05). Recovery of hunger is rapid after small meals and no significant differences are present in size of the first bout of second meals between any of the intervals used. After medium-sized meals significant differences exist between all combinations of intervals apart from 24 and 48 hrs (M-W U test, p< 0,05). Both of these approached closely the mean 1st bout length for first meals in Experiment 1 (15.4 s). Significant differences were present between all inter-meal intervals used after large meals (M-W U test, p< 0.05) indicating that hunger was not fully recovered after 48 hrs. This is in agreement with the results of Experiment 1.

Pathogen survival in H. irritans

The survival of mixed cultures of *C. pyogenes* and *P. indolicus* in *H. irritans* (Exp. 4) under the conditions used in this experiment is given in Fig. 1 for each pathogen separately. Both *C. pyogenes* and *P. indolicus* could be recovered from the vector for at least 4 days after a full meal and 3 days after an interrupted meal although there were indications that *P. indolicus* was also present 7 days after a full meal. The decrease in number of c.f.u.'s recovered is not completely linear, particularly as far as *C. pyogenes* is concerned, where it even appears to increase between 12 and 24 hrs.

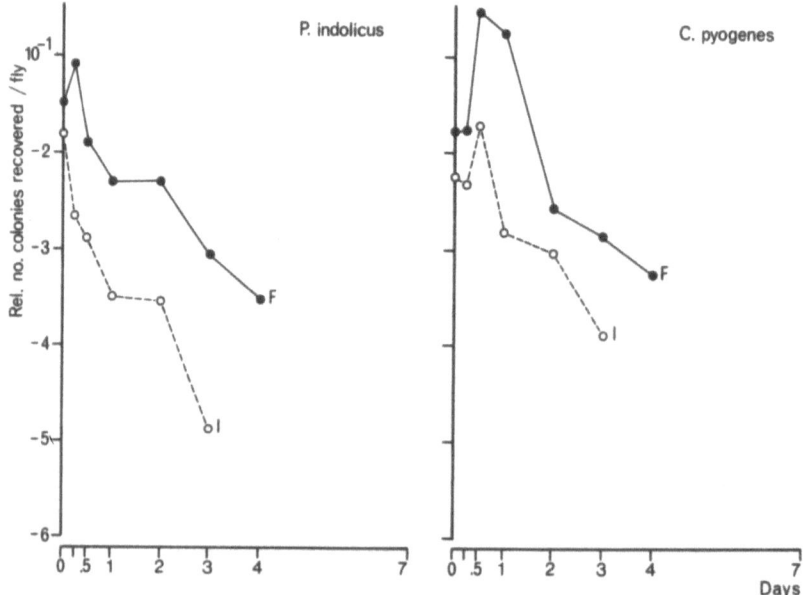

Fig. 1. Relative number of colonies recovered from *H. irritans* as a function of time after feeding a mixture of *C. pyogenes* and *P. indolicus*. (F = full meal; I = interrupted meal).

bacterially 'spiced' meal. The BHI droplet was then plated and incubated in the same way as in Exp. 4 except that no dilution series was made. The clearly identifiable fly faeces were dissolved and removed using a loop and 0.02 ml of BHI and incubated in the same way.

RESULTS

Feeding motivation

The results of experiments 1 and 2 are given in Table 1. The mean durations of the first bouts and total proboscis contact for meal 1 of the serum/serum experiment were 15 and 106.7 s, respectively. For the serum/blood experiment these figures were 15.4 and 89.6 s. Given that the fly feeds on the same substrate, it appears that an interval of at least 4 days is necessary for feeding motivation to recover completely. In the serum/blood experiment however, no clear trends in relation to inter-meal interval are present but blood meals are generally longer than the first serum meal.

TABLE 1.　Recovery of hunger expressed as the mean difference in feeding motivation (Δ in s) in first bout and total proboscis contact time between successive meals in relation to the duration of inter-meal interval.

Substrate	Behaviour measured	Interval between 1st and 2nd meal in days 1	2	3	4
Serum/Serum	Δ 1st bout	−10.10	− 2.60	−13.30	+ 0.88
Serum/Serum	Δ total meal	−63.20	−46.50	−57.80	−39.80
Serum/Blood	Δ 1st bout	+ 8.70	− 9.30	+15.00	+ 5.30
Serum/Blood	Δ total meal	+ 16.30	+74.80	+28.80	− 4.90

TABLE 2.　Mean duration of the first bout of the 2nd meal in seconds after different inter-meal intervals for small (5 s), medium (25 s) and long (50 s) first meals.

Duration of 1st meal	Interval between the two meals in hrs 6	12	24	48
Small	7.9	9.4	16.7	16.7
Medium	5.7	11.8	14.0	16.8
Large	1.9	10.9	11.7	10.1

The effect of manipulating the duration of a meal on recovery of hunger is shown in Table 2.

Fig. 2 gives the equivalent data for Exp. 5 after feeding monocultures of the pathogenes. *Streptococcus dysgalactiae* appears to remain stable for the first 24 hrs. Unfortunately, all flies died at this point and no further data could be collected. The survival of *P. indolicus* corresponds to that in Experiment 4, but that of *C. pyogenes* differs completely when fed as a monoculture. No decrease occurs in the number of c.f.u.'s recovered during the time the experiment was run.

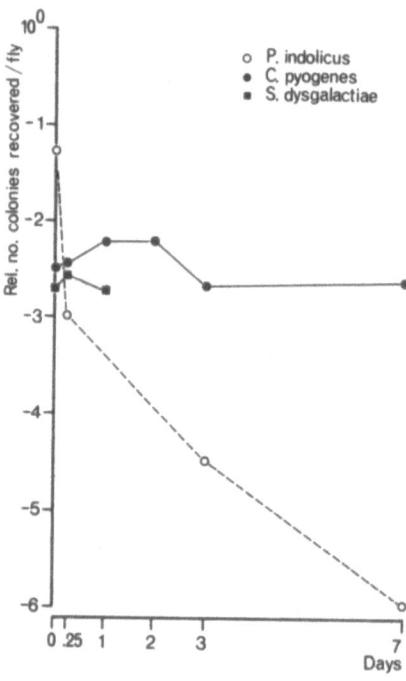

Fig. 2. Relative number of colonies recovered from *H. irritans* as a function of time after feeding monocultures of *C. pyogenes, P. indolicus* and *S. dysgalactiae.*

In vitro transmission of pathogens via H. irritans

The results of Experiment 6 are summarized in Table 3. The following points may be made regarding bacterial transmission under the conditions used in the experiment. Firstly, recovery of *C. pyogenes* from subsequent meals appears to be very poor except when the interval is 0. The same applies to *P. indolicus* although this can be transmitted over longer time intervals. As far as recovery from faeces is concerned, fairly high numbers of *P. indolicus* c.f.u.'s were recovered 24 hrs after feeding on the bacterial meal.

TABLE 3. Number of c.f.u.'s recovered from subsequent meals and faeces as a function of time. The data for full and interrupted bacterially 'spiced' meals are given separately. (P.i. = *P. indolicus*, C.p. = *C. pyogenes*; (N) = No. of flies)

Interval in hrs	No. c.f.u.'s recovered from									
	Meal						Faeces			
	Full			Interrupted			Full		Interrupted	
	P.i.	C.p.	(N)	P.i.	C.p.	(N)	P.i.	C.p.	P.i.	C.p.
0	>300	>300	(20)	>300	>300	(20)	0	0	0	0
1	70	0	(20)	96	0	(20)	0	0	1	3
6	9	0	(20)	3	0	(20)	0	0	0	0
24	1	0	(15)	7	0	(13)	2	0	73	0
96	4	0	(12)	0	0	(6)	0	0	0	0

DISCUSSION

As far as feeding motivation is concerned the results indicate that at least 4 days are required for hunger to recover completely after *H. irritans* is allowed to feed to repletion on a protein meal. If the fly is only provided with a short meal (5 s) this period is very much shorter and recovery will occur within 24 hrs. The duration of a meal will not only depend on the interval from the preceding meal it will also depend on the substrate being fed upon as is shown by Exp. 3. It has been shown that meal duration is positively correlated with the viscosity of the substrate (Nielsen and Madsen, 1985). Although the defibrinated blood used for the 2nd meals in Exp. 2 will certainly have a higher viscosity than the serum used for the 1st meals this factor alone is not sufficient to explain lack of trend found in recovery of hunger. In all probability taste and/or quality variables are involved which act as positive feedbacks and increase hunger (Thomas, 1976).

As far as the experiments on bacterial survival in the vector are concerned, both *C. pyogenes* and *P. indolicus* could be recovered for between 4 and 7 days. Moreover, even when *H. irritans* is only allowed a short feeding period (10 s) considerable numbers of these bacteria survive in the fly for at least 3 days. Wright and Titchener (1977) were able to recover *C. pyogenes* for a much longer period than found in Exp. 4 (>16 days). The results of Exp. 5 however, offers a possible explanation for this. When fed as a monoculture – the procedure followed by Wright and Titchener – *C. pyogenes* survived at a constant level for at least 7 days. This suggests that interactions occur between *C. pyogenes* and *P. indolicus* when these are simultaneously present within *H. irritans*. Laboratory experiments have demonstrated that the two pathogens do interact (Sorensen, 1980) in that *P. indolicus* stimulates the growth of *C. pyogenes*. The results found here however, suggest that the interactions between these pathogens within the fly are different and it may well be that

P. indolicus inhibits *C. pyogenes* in this particular environment.

The results of Experiment 6 demonstrates that *H. irritans* can imbibe two of the pathogenes implicated in summer mastitis and deposit these on another substrate at a later period of time. This may occur via feeding behaviour but transmission via fly faeces is also a possibility. More success was achieved with *P. indolicus* than with *C. pyogenes*. However, in experiments carried out in 1985 (Thomas and Hillerton, unpubl. results), not only was successful transmission of *C. pyogenes* obtained using *H. irritans* but the interval between bacterial uptake and deposition was at least 2 days. Moreover, Madsen and Sorensen (1985) were able to achieve transmission of both bacteria after an interval of 7 days. Obviously a great deal remains to be done in this area. One striking difference between the three success-ful artificial transmission attempts described above is the fact that the sterile substrate used as a second meal differed. In the experiment described here use was made of BHI, in the experiments with Hillerton we used full blood which was allowed to clot. Finally, Madsen and Sorensen used solid blood/agar. Like all sucking muscid flies, *H. irritans* modifies its method of feeding depending on the substrate (Dethier, 1976). The more solid this is, the greater the tendancy for the fly to regurgitate liquid onto the substrate to make this more fluid. This habit could well result in depositing higher bacterial loads as suggested by Hillerton and Thomas (1985) and could explain the differences found in transmission interval between the experiments.

ACKNOWLEDGEMENTS

We wish to thank the National Animal Health Committee, the Hague and the Central Veterinary Institute for supporting the research.

A CULTURE TECHNIQUE FOR HYDROTAEA IRRITANS

H.J. Over, G. Thomas, J.N. van der Linden, M.J. van den Berg and A. van der Lugt

Central Veterinary Institute
P.O. Box 65, 8200 AB Lelystad, The Netherlands

ABSTRACT

One of the major disadvantages in carrying out research on *H. irritans* is the lack of a reliable culture technique for this fly species.

Previous attempts to culture the sheep headfly only resulted in a very low production of adult flies.

In order to carry out sensory physiology and behavioural tests and to ensure well defined and bacteriologically "clean" flies a reliable culture technique is a prerequisite.

Experiments were done to determine the oviposition habitat and to ensure high larval survival, pupation rate and fly emergence.

Diet and holding temperature clearly influenced all three parameters giving with *Enchytraeus* and 15°C a pupation percentage of 62.5 and a fly emergence of 38.5%.

As yet, despite several attempts, no successful copulations have been obtained.

1. INTRODUCTION

Attempts to culture *H. irritans* in the laboratory are economically justified by the association of this fly species and broken heads in sheep and because of its probable role in the transmission of summer mastitis.

There are three fields of interest that have evoked the attempts to cultivate *H. irritans*.

Firstly, cultivation of the fly gives insight into the general biology of the species and the observations are of primary importance for the causal analysis of the phenomena met in the field situation. In the latter respect, the original work of Overgaard Nielsen *et al.* (1971), Tarry and Kirkwood (1976), Robinson (1979), Berlyn (1979) and Ball *et al.* (1985) have increased our knowledge considerably.

Secondly, sensory physiology and behavioural studies benefit much from a reliable culture method as the value of conclusions in these fields of investigation is highly dependent on the continuous availability of well defined and consistent biological material. This was in fact our goal in starting and improving a *Hydrotaea* culture during the last few years. Moreover it was realized that in order to perform transmission trials, standardized adult flies with consistent characteristics might be of importance: The third objective.

As we implicitly believe that control of the diseases mentioned above has to be based upon a rather subtle kind of manipulation of the vector/pathogen and vector-host contacts we explicitly concentrated our interest on efforts to culture *H. irritans* in the laboratory in order to get a constant source of eggs, larvae and adults over a longer period than the field situation can provide.

2. LOGISTICS

In the life cycle of Diptera the transition rates between four phases should be distinguished:

1. eggs
2. 1st, 2nd and 3rd instar larvae
3. pupae
4. imago's.

As in *H. irritans* first instar larvae are already contained within the egg and the transition via the 2nd stage to the third is easy, the following items are analyzed in this paper:

1. Induction of oviposition.
2. Survival of larvae.
3. Induction of pupation.
4. Survival of pupae.
5. Induction of emergence.
6. Survival of the flies.
7. Induction of copulation.

The combination of reliable induction and high survival phases is the characteristic of a successful culture method.

3. THE DIFFERENT PHASES:

3.1. *Induction of oviposition.*

For reasons to be mentioned in 3.7 our data only refer to female flies hand captured in the field. Stimulation of oviposition is not difficult (Overgaard Nielsen *et al*, 1971; Kirkwood, 1976; Robinson and Luff, 1976; Berlyn, 1979). Depending upon the season, inseminated females are easily collected in the field in the period August-September and on a variety of simple diets will survive and oviposit for some months.

Just as in their experiments, females will oviposit on almost any substrate given sufficient moisture. Petri dishes containing peat, leaf litter, soil or cow dung or mixtures of these in the cages act as oviposition sites. In comparative trials, pure wet sand or peat soil proved to be an inferior site. At the moment in our laboratory, oviposition sites are simulated by introducing small, semi-open, moist, grass tufts with litter and sandy profiles into the holding cages (Plate 1-A). Incidentally, the water-saturated cotton plug in the top of the cage not only provided a source of moisture for the flies but was used a successful oviposition site as well. Cages were placed inside at 20°C but under natural daylight.

3.2. *Survival of larvae.*

The 2nd instar larvae (7 ds) are collected by hand washing from the turf. The individual larvae are transferred by means of a paint-brush to the larval habitats *i.e.* small tubes filled with a peat-leaf litter mixture (Plate 1-B, left).

Although involving a high labor-investment, keeping them individually is necessary as communal housing greatly impairs the transition rate (Table 1) as is shown in the daily mortality because of cannibalism.

Keeping them individually we fed them different menus. Three times a week feeding resulted in the data presented in Table 2. In our experience the mixed food (*D. melanogaster-*, Tipulid-larvae, *Lucilia ceasar-*, *Rhizopertha dominica* larvae and *Enchytraeus*) or exclusively feeding them with *Enchytraeus* induced the most favourable results in terms of pupation and emergence.

With regard to the culture temperature, 15°C proved to be superior to 21°C (Table 3) as might be anticipated in relation to the situation in the field. We have recently initiated observations at 12°C.

TABLE 1. Effect of housing on larval mortality

		N larvae at start (Ns)	N larvae at end (Ne)	N days (D)	Mortality
Communal housing	1	55	31	20	2.18
	2	58	17	18	3.90
	3	23	8	12	5.44
	4	131	48	12	5.28
Individual housing	1	31	15	46	1.12
	2	17	14	46	0.38
	3	8	6	46	0.54
	4	48	44	38	0.22

Daily mortality defined as $\{[(Ns-Ne)/Ns]/D\}$ 100.

TABLE 2. Effect of diet on pupation and emergence

	DR	DR+ENCH	DR+TIP	DR+RD	DR+LUC	MIX	ENCH
N start	91	91	91	91	91	182	91
% Pupae	20.8	23.8	21.4	32.3	35.9	47.4	62.5
% Flies	5.5	5.5	6.6	12.1	18.7	29.7	38.5

———— Equals n.s. level (5%).

3.3. *Induction of pupation.*

From the work of the authors mentioned above it is clear that after some months of growing, 3rd instar larvae (Plate 1-C) cease eating. This inactive phase starts in the field in

November and finishes in pupation sometime late in spring. In the field it is assumed that this occurs in May (Robinson, 1979).

In attempts to break down this resting phase we manipulated the larval breeding temperature (15°C) in different ways. Lowering the temperature to 5°C did not induce pupation but preliminary data show that a subsequent temperature rise to 21°C might do so (Table 4). At the moment we are running an experiment in order to see if this shock might result in pupation at earlier moments during the resting phase of the larvae as well.

TABLE 3. Effect of temperature on pupation and emergence

	N start	N pupae (%)	N flies emerging (%)
21°C	100	1 (1)	0 (0)
15°C	719	318 (44.2)	133 (18.5)
Outside (Oct-May)	100	? (?)	12 (12.0)

TABLE 4. Effect of warm shock on pupation

	N larvae 8/4	N pupae 1/5	N flies 1/5
15 − 21°C	28	18	4
15°C continuous	35	4	0

3.4—5. *Survival of the pupae and emergence.*

Pupae run the risk of drying out or being infected by fungi if the habitat is too wet. After collection of the pupae from the larval culture tubes they are transferred to ones filled with a more sandy mixture. Depending upon the temperature the imagoes will emerge (Plate 1-D) after 2-5 wks.

The pupae tubes are provided with a cap that makes early drinking by the flies after emergence possible (Plate 1-B, right).

3.6—7. *Survival of the flies and copulation.*

Flies are kept in perspex or polyethylene covered cages at 18°C on a 16—8 L/D regime. Continuous feeding with a 5% sucrose-solution via a saturated cotton-wool plug is necessary (Plate 1-E).

Dead flies should be removed. For the analysis of copulation behaviour, sexes should be kept apart from emergence onward.

In order to induce copulation we tried different feeding substrates for male and female,

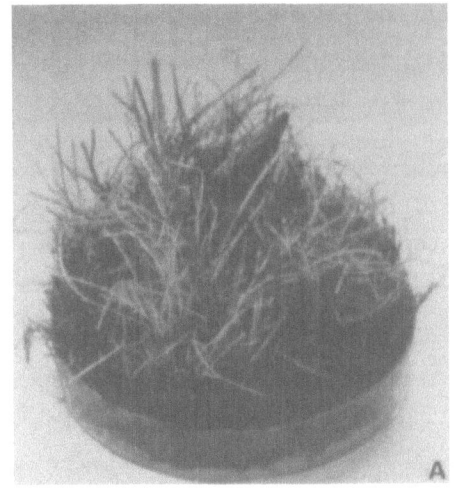

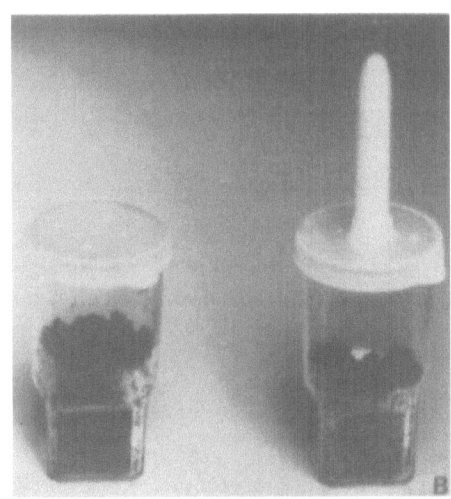

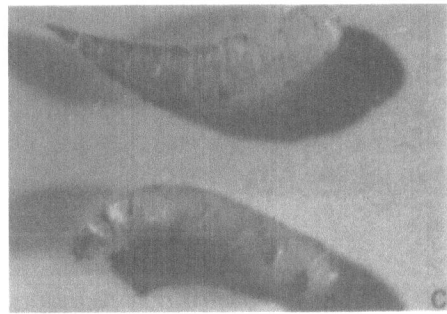

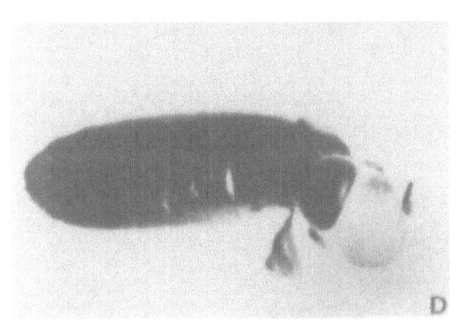

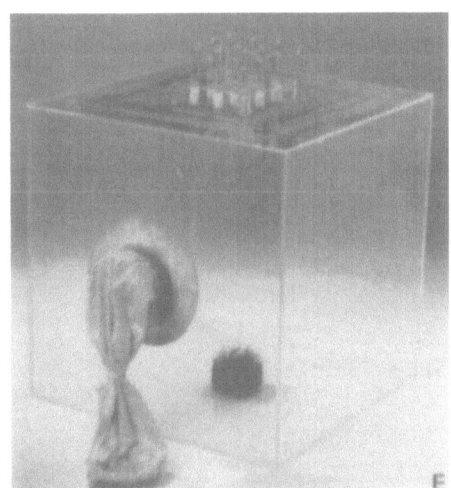

Plate I-A Method for offering oviposition substrate.
" I-B Individual culture (left) and emergence tubes (right).
" I-C Full grown larva of *H. irritans*.
" I-D Adult fly emergence from pupa.
" I-E Holding cages showing feeding tubes.

manipulated the copulation environments but until now we have been unsuccessful. Next year more trials with regard to this aspect are planned in other experimental situations.

4. CONCLUSION:

At the moment with regard to survival of eggs, larvae and pupae in our set up we have been rather successful. With regard to speeding up the transition the results are merely indicative as far as pupation and emergence are concerned. The induction of copulation still offers a problem of bewildering possibilities. In order to realize a reliable culture technique, producing the different stages over the year, these problems have to be solved, the last one in particular. Summarizing our data at the moment results in the following list of culture conditions for *H. irritans.*

Eggs   Substrate   : Natural sandy profile
                                     open grasstufts
              Temp.   : 21°C 7 − 10 ds
              Humidity   : 90% approx.

Larvae   Substrate   : Peat-leaf litter mixture
              Temp.   : 15°C 17 wks
              Humidity   : not water saturated, not dry
              Food   : Enchytraeus ± 1 cm: 3 times/wk
              Individual housing.

Pupae   Substrate   : as Larvae but more sandy
              Temp.   : 15°C 24 − 36 ds
                                     21°C 14 − 21 ds
              Humidity   : see Larvae.

Flies   Cage   : "soft surfaces", no wire gauze
              Temp.   : 18°C some mths
              Humidity   : 65%
              Food   : water resp. 5% sucrose solution
                                     Defibrinized cattle blood.

REFERENCES

Aehnelt, E. von. 1955. Zur Vorbeuge der Pyogenes-Mastitis bei Weiderindern mit Kontakt-insektiziden. DTW., **62**, 493-498.

Anon. 1942. The control of certain diseases in dairy cows. Vet. Rec., **54**, 194.

Bahr, L. 1952. Some investigations on "Summer mastitis". 1. Dansk Maanedsskr. Dyrl., **62**, 367-394. (In Danish, English summary).

Bahr, L. 1955. Fortsatte undersogelser vedrorende "sommermastitis" hos goldkvaeget. Anden meddelese. Dansk. Manedsskr. Dyrl., **63**, 365-388.

Ball, S.G. 1984. Seasonal abundance during the summer months of some cattle visiting Muscidae (Diptera) in north-east England. Ecol. Entomol., **9**, 1-10.

Ball, S.G., Port, G.R. and Luff, M.L. 1985. Aspects of the reproductive biology of some cattle visiting Muscidae (Diptera) in north-east England. Vet. Par., **18**, 183-196.

Berlyn, A.D. 1979. The effect of diet on the life span and egg maturation of caged adult sheep headflies *Hydrotaea irritans* (Fallén) (Diptera: Muscidae). Bull ent. Res., **69**, 299-307.

Bramley, A.J., Hillerton, J.E., Higgs, T.M. and Hogben, E.M. 1985. The carriage of summer mastitis pathogens by muscid flies. Br. vet. J., **141**, 618-627.

Campbell, D. 1941. Bovine mastitis. Vet. Rec., **53**, 755.

Colwell, R.K. and Futuyma, D.J. 1971. On the measurement of niche breadth and overlap. Ecol., **52**, 567-576.

Chvála, M., Lyneborg, L. and Moucha, J. 1972. The horse flies of Europe. (Diptera, Tabanidae). Entomol. Soc. Copenhagen.

Dethier, V.G. 1976. The Hungry Fly. Harvard University Press, Cambridge (Mass.) and London (U.K.).

Elger, D. 1985. Untersuchungen zur Biologie und Ökologie symboviner Musciden und Tabaniden in Norddeutschland (Diptera: Muscidae, Tabanidae). Thesis, Hannover.

Elger, D. and Liebisch, A. 1982. Felduntersuchungen zur Wirksamkeit von Permethrin zur Bekämpfung von Fliegen an Weiderindern in Norddeutschland. Tierärztl. Umschau **37**, 437-442.

Francis, J. 1941. A bacteriological examination of bovine tonsils and vaginas. The possible relationship of the findings to mastitis and pneumonia. Br. Vet. J., **97**, 243-251.

Frydenberg, O. and Simonsen, V. 1973. Genetics of *Zoarces* populations. V. Amount of protein polymorphism and degree of genetic heterozygosity. Hereditas, **75**, 221-232.

Giesecke, W.H. 1985. The effect of stress on udder health of dairy cows. Onderstepoort J. Vet. Res., **52**, 175-193.

Hammer, O. 1941. Biological and ecological investigations on flies associated with pasturing cattle and their excrement. Vidensk. Medd. Dansk naturh. Foren., **105**, 141-393.

Hansen, J. and Nielsen, S.A. 1983. Summermastitis: a review. Heifer Mastitis Seminar, Stockholm-Helsinki.

Hennig, W. 1964. Muscidae. In: E. Lindner, Ed. Die Fliegen der palaearktischen Region. Vol. VII, part 1 and 2. Schweizerbartsche Verlagsbuchhandlung, Stuttgart.

Hillerton, J.E. Bramley, A.J. and Broom. D.M. 1983. *Hydrotaea irritans* and summer mastitis in calves. Vet. Rec., **113**, 88.

Hillerton, J.E. and Bramley, A.J. 1985. Carriage of *Corynebacterium pyogenes* by the cattle nuisance flies *Hydrotaea irritans* (Fall.) and *Musca autumnalis* (DeG.). Vet. Par., **18**, 223-228.

Hillerton, J.E. and Thomas, G. 1986. Transmission of summer mastitis by flies. Abstr. 1st Int. Cong. Dipterology, (ed. B. Dasvas and L. Papp.) Budapest. p. 95.

Horvath, D.J. and Reid, R.L. 1984. Indirect effects of soil and water on animal health. Sci. Tot. Envir., **34**, 143-156.

Hucket, H.C. 1954. A review of the North American species belonging to the genus Hydrotaea Robineau-Desvoidy (Diptera: Muscidae). Ann. Entomol. Soc. Amer., **47**, 316-342.

Jones, R.N. and Rees, H. 1982. B-chromosomes. Academic Press, New York.

Jonsson, P., Olsson, S-O., Holmberg, O. and Funke, H. 1986. Heifer mastitis in Sweden during a three-year-period (1982-1985). Bacteriological findings in udder secretion from clinical and subclinical cases. Proc. "EEC workshop on summer mastitis", 23-24 Oct. 1986, Lelystad, The Netherlands.

Kirkwood, A.C. 1976. Ovarian and larval development of the sheep headfly, *Hydrotaea irritans* (Fallén) (Diptera: Muscidae). Bull. Ent. Res., **66**, 757-763.

Kirkwood, A.C. and Tarry, D.W. 1973. A survey of some species of flies associated with cattle. Int. Pest Contr., **15**, 6-10.

Liebisch, A. and Elger, D. 1983. Weidefliegen und deren Bekämpfung bei Rindern. Fortschr. Veterinärmed. Heft 37: 15. Kongressbericht, 267.

Lindner, E. 1949. Die Fliegen der palaearktischen Region. Vol. 1. Schweizerbartsche Verslagsbuchhandlung, Stuttgart.

Loeschke, V. and Christensen. B. 1986. Variation in chromosome number in the sheep headfly *Hydrotaea irritans* (Fallen) (Diptera: Muscidae). Experientia, in press.

Lovell, R. 1943. The source of *Corynebacterium pyogenes* infections. Vet. Rec., **55**, 99-100.

Lovell, R. 1945. *Corynebacterium pyogenes* infections of domestic animals. Vet. Rec., **57**, 683-685.

Madsen, M. 1985. Summer mastitis. Thesis. Royal Veterinary and Agricultural University, Copenhagen. (In Danish, English summary).

Madsen, M. and Sorensen, G. Hoi. 1985. Transmissionsdynamiske aspekter vedrorende spredning af "sommermastitis-bakterier" med dipterer. In "Initiativet: Sommermastitis", ed. P. Nansen. (Report to the Danish Agricultural and Veterinary Research Council, Copenhagen.)

Madsen, M., Nielsen, S.A. and Nansen, P. 1986. Summer mastitis. Presentation of a 4-year reserach project. Dansk Vet. Tidsskr., **69**, 533-543. (In Danish).

Mair, K.-H. 1980. Das Vorkommen von Dipteren an Jungrindern auf Bergweiden im Bayrischen Allgäu. Vet. med. Thesis, Munich.

Marshall, A.B. 1981. Summer mastitis. Technical Bulletin 4. N.I.R.D., Reading, U.K. and Hannah Res. Inst. Ayr. Scott.

Mayer, K. 1981. Untersuchungen über das Vorkommen von Dipteren an Weiderindern und die Verbreitung von Zecken im Bayrischen Allgäu. Vet. med. Thesis, Munich.

McEwen, A.D. 1942. Notes concerning abortion, mastitis and sterility. Vet. Rec., **54**, 155.

Michael, L. 1983. Untersuchungen symboviner Fliegen auf *Corynebacterium pyogenes* unter besonderer Berücksichtigung der Sommermastitis. Vet. med. Thesis, Hannover.

Moucha, J. and Chvála, M. 1968. Die Gattung Hybomitra Enderlein, 1922 in der Tschechoslowakei (Diptera: Tabanidae). Act. faun. ent. Mus. nat. Prague, **12**, 263-294.

Nansen, P. 1985. ed. "Initiativet: Sommermastitis", (Report to the Danish Agricultural and Veterinary Research Council, Copenhagen).

Natterman, H. von and Horsch, F. 1976. Zur Pathogenese der *Corynebacterium-pyogenes*-Mastitis des Rindes. Monatsch. Vet.-med., **32**, 342-345.

Nielsen, S.A. and Madsen, M. 1985. Status over fourageringsaktiviteten hos plantagefluen (*Hydrotaea irritans* Fall.) med saerlig henblik pa praeferens for forskellige fourageringsmedier. In "Initiativet: Sommermastitis", ed. P. Nansen. (Report to the Danish Agricultural and Veterinary Research Council, Copenhagen).

Nielsen, S.A., Jespersen, J.B., Bjorn, H. and Nielsen, B. Overgaard. 1985a. The composition of the fauna of Diptera on pasturing cattle in Denmark. In "Sommer mastitis" (Ed. P. Nansen). (Report to the Danish Agricultural and Veterinary Research Council, Copenhagen). pp 168-180.

Nielsen, S.A., Jespersen, J.B. and Nielsen, B. Overgaard. 1985b. Distribution of Diptera over the bodies of pasturing cattle. In "Sommer mastitis" (Ed. P. Nansen). (Report to the Danish Agricultural and Veterinary Research Council, Copenhagen), pp. 181-198.

Nielsen, S.A., Nielsen, B. Overgaard, Hansen, J.W., Nansen, P. and Olesen, J. 1985c. Fourageringsaktivitet hos *Hydrotaea irritans* i relation til klimaet. In "Initiativet: Sommermastitis", ed. P. Nansen. (Report to the Danish Agricultural and Veterinary Research Council, Copenhagen).

Nielsen, B. Overgaard, Moller-Nielsen, B. and Christensen, O. 1971. Bidrag til plantagefluens, *Hydrotaea irritans* (Fall.) (Diptera: Muscidae) biologi. Ent. Meddr., **39**, 30-44.

Nielsen, B. Overgaard, Moller-Nielsen, B. and Christensen, O. 1972. Plantagefluen, *Hydrotaea irritans* (Fall.) (Diptera: Muscidae) på graessende kvier. Ent. Meddr., **40**, 151-173.

Olesen, J.E., Nielsen, S.A., Hansen, J.W. and Nansen, P. 1985. Sommermastitis. Incidens, tidspunkt for optraeden m.m. i relation til klima i observationsperioden 1953-1981. In "Initiativet: Sommermastitis", ed. P. Nansen. (Report to the Danish Agricultural and Veterinary Research Council, Copenhagen).

Olsson, S-O., Jonsson, P., Holmberg, O. and Funke, H. 1986. Heifer mastitis in Sweden during a trhee-year-period (1982-1985). Background and some preliminary data on the incidence of heifer mastitis. Proc. "EEC workshop on summer mastitis", 23-24 Oct. 1986, Lelystad, The Netherlands.

Peus, F. 1980. Über Bremsen aus der westlichen Paläarktis. Dtsch. Ent. Z., **27**, 221-249.

Radola, B.J. 1980 Ultrathin-layer isoelectric focusing in 50-100 μm polyacrylamide gels on silanized glass plates or polyester films. Electrophoresis, **1**, 43-56.

Robinson, J. 1979. The sheep headfly, *Hydrotaea irritans* (Fallén) (Diptera: Muscidae): biology of the immature stages in the soil. Bull. Ent. Res., **69**. 589-598.

Robinson, J. and Luff, M.L. 1976. The sheep headfly, *Hydrotaea irritans* (Fallén) (Diptera: Muscidae): larval habitat and immature stages. Bull. Ent. Res., **65**, 579-586.

Saes, J.M.F. 1970. Voorkomen, pathogenese en bestrijding van *Corynebacterium pyogenes* mastitis (Wrang) bij runderen in Limburg. Thesis, Utrecht.

Skidmore, P. 1985. "The Biology of the Muscidae of the World" Dr. W. Junk Publ. Dordrecht, Boston, Lancaster.

Sorensen, G. Hoi. 1974. Studies on the aetiology and transmission of summer mastitis. Nord. Vet.-Med., **26**, 122-133.

Sorensen, G. Hoi. 1976. Studies on the occurrence of *Peptococcus indolicus* and *Corynebacterium pyogenes* in apparently healthy cattle. Act. Vet. Scand., **17**, 15-24.

Sorensen, G. Hoi. 1978. Bacteriological examination of summer mastitis secretions. The demonstration of Bacteroidaceae. Nord. Vet. Med., **30**, 199-204.

Sorensen, G. Hoi. 1980. Comparative studies on *Corynebacterium pyogenes* toxin formation in monocultures and mixed cultures - the demonstration of a stimulating effect of *Peptococcus indolicus* and Stuart-Schwan cocci. Act. Vet. Scand., **21**, 438-448.

Stein, M., Keller, S.E. and Schleifer, S.J. 1985. Stress and immunomodulation: the role of depression and neuroendocrine function. J. Immunol., **35**, 827-833.

Stuart, P., Buntain, D. and Langridge, R.G. 1951. Bacteriological examinations of secretions from cases of "Summer Mastitis" and experimental infections of non-lactating bovine udders. Vet. Rec., **63**, 451-453.

Stuart, P. and Parish, W.E. 1955. HMSO Report on the Animal Health Services in Great Britain.

Stuart, P. and Parish, W.E. 1956. HMSO Report on the Animal Health Services in Great Britain.

Tarry, D.W. 1975. The significance of feeding and blood meal identification studies in the planning of sheep headfly control measures. Proc. 8th Br. Insecticide and Fungicide Conf., 573-580.

Tarry, D.W. and Kirkwood, A.C. 1976. Biology and development of the sheep headfly *Hydrotaea irritans* (Fall) (Diptera: Muscidae). Bull. Ent. Res., **65**, 587-594.

Tarry, D.W., Wilson, C.D. and Stuart, P. 1978. The headfly *Hydrotaea irritans* and summer mastitis infection. Vet. Rec., **102**, 91.

Thomas, G. 1976. Gust and disgust or the causes of alliesthesia. Thesis, Groningen.

Thomas, G., Schomaker, C.H., Been, T.H., v.d. Berg, M.J. and Prijs, H.J. 1985. Host finding and feeding in *Hydrotaea irritans* (Diptera: Muscidae): The role of chemical senses. Vet. Par., **18**, 209-221.

Titchener, R.N., Newbold, J.W. and Wright, C.L. 1981. Flies associated with cattle in South West Scotland during the summer months. Res. Vet. Sci., **30**, 109-113.

Tolle, A., Franke, V. and Reichmuth, J. 1983. Zur *C. pyogenes*-Mastitis. Bakteriologische Aspekte. DTW, **90**, 256-260.

Wright, C.L. and Titchener, R.N. 1977. Infection of the sheep headfly, *Hydrotaea irritans* with bacterial isolates from field cases of summer mastitis. Vet. Rec., **101**, 426.

Ziegler, E. 1970. Untersuchungen zur Fliegenfauna an Rindern in Stallungen und auf der Weide. Vet. med. Thesis, Humboldt Univ. Berlin.

Zumpt, F. 1973. The Stomoxine biting flies on the world. Diptera: Muscidae. Gustav Fischer Verlag, Stuttgart.

DISCUSSION

The discussion centered on three general areas.

(a) Transmission experiments.

(b) Interactions between symbovine dipterans.

(c) Genetic variability within *H. irritans* in relation to vector function.

The discussion on the first point centered on possibilities for resolving the difficulty experienced by several groups in attempting to replicate the successful *in vivo* transmission experiments carried out at Weybridge in the 50's and 70's using *Hydrotaea irritans* as a vector for summer mastitis pathogens. There was a general consensus in the need to continue experiments on survival and transmission dynamics of summer mastitis pathogens within the fly as this information is essential for improving the design of experiments. Furthermore, the suggestion was put forward that the experimental models applied to date generally made use of that category of animals — non-pregnant heifers — which did not give the most optimal probability of successful infection. It was proposed that, given the data presented by Hillerton in Section I regarding the relative incidence of summer mastitis in different age and pregnancy categories, future attempts should make use of pregnant, dry cows as this is the highest risk group. Opinions were then exchanged regarding the pros and cons of using this category of animals. One possible negative aspect brought up was the fact that spontaneous, endogenously originating infection may occur due to physiological stress during drying off even in the absence of flies. This could invalidate any conclusions from a fly transmission experiment. The discussion continued with the suggestion that spontaneous mastitis infections in dry cows during the summer rarely involve summer mastitis pathogens which would reduce the objection against using such animals. In fact consideration should be given to the possibility that such dry cow mastitis infections act as a predisposing factor for fly transmitted infections with summer mastitis pathogens. This part of the discussion was closed with a remark from the floor that the circumstantial evidence supporting fly transmission was so strong that success in transmission experiments was not all that crucial.

Following this, the point was raised that some of the other symbovine dipterans have a similar activity pattern and site selection on the host to *Hydrotaea irritans*. The question was phrased whether any possibilities existed regarding interactions between these species and *H. irritans* in the transmission process, particularly in biting insects providing potential feeding places. Information on the German situation indicated a coincidence between the pattern of seasonal activity of Tabanids and *H. irritans*, moreover some of the former species show the same feeding site preference. However, it was pointed out that the number of Tabanids is rather low in England and Denmark and, although there is one species commonly found on the teat in the latter country, the general consensus of the researchers in these two regions was that Tabanid species do not play a critical role. In Denmark, interactions are potentially possible between *H. irritans* and the biting midges (Ceratopogonidae) and blackflies (Simuliidae) some of which leave wounds and damage the teat and udder epidermis. It was remarked that in England there is a temporal discontiguity as far as biting midges are concerned as these are predominantly active at dusk when *H. irritans* activity has stopped. However, this did not negate the possibility of interaction as the lesions remaining could provide a secondary feeding site and source of attraction for *H. irritans*. It appeared that in Germany biting midges forage more dorsally on the host body where thousands may be present in the hair covered areas. Finally, a question was raised as to the possibility of interaction between the horn fly *Haematobia irritans* and *Hydrotaea irritans*. The general consensus of the entomologists was that horn flies rarely feed on the udder and teat and are not likely to interact with *H. irritans* by *e.g.* providing potential feeding sites.

In designing *in vivo* transmission experiments, teat damage caused by biting insects is often simulated using sterile needles before allowing infected *H. irritans* access to the organ. It was indicated that the primary damage left by biting insects will differ in several aspects to damage left by a needle because there is often a local reaction to bites. The general consensus was that there was a paucity of information on insect interactions but that these could possibly play a role in the transmission process and thus require more emphasis in future research.

Finally, the potential relevance of studies into chromosome and enzyme variation in *H. irritans* for transmission of summer mastitis was discussed. It was pointed out that studies of other insect vectors of disease *e.g.* mosquitoes showed that several species, subspecies, biotypes *etc.* exist which not only differ very much in biology but also in vector capacity. Whether the same in true for *H. irritans* remains to be determined but there are arguments suggesting this possibility.

5. PREVENTION AND THERAPY

Chairmen J. Sol & A. Liebisch

THE PREVENTION AND THERAPY OF SUMMER MASTITIS IN EUROPE

J. Sol

Animal Health Service Institute in Overijssel and Flevoland,
Postbus 13, 8000 AA Zwolle, The Netherlands.

ABSTRACT

There are several methods of preventing summer mastitis. Long acting antibiotics and ear-tags containing insecticides are the most effective. Administration of long acting antibiotics protects almost completely for four weeks. Ear-tags also provide a good protection for up to 3 to 4 months. Although the incidence of summer mastitis is low, cases are still seen but are almost independent of the time after applying ear-tags. Bacteriological examination of the latter cases turned up mostly bacteria which are not typical for summer mastitis. The best choice for preventing summer mastitis in dry cows are long acting antibiotics and in heifers, ear-tags. A dry cow treatment has to be repeated after 4 weeks.

Treatment of summer mastitis is usually unsuccessful in saving the udder tissue especially if there is systemic illness, a hard swollen quarter and the typical odour. Surgical removal of the teat is not advisable. It is important for prognosis, particularly in dry cows, to take a sample for bacteriological examination. Therapy is usually successful in restoring general health. In general, cows are most sick. A summer mastitis case has to be separated from the herd. After detecting a case, the remainder of the herd must be watched very closely for the next few days. When this is done new cases will be detected in about 35% of the herds, almost independent of the herd size.

THE PREVENTION OF SUMMER MASTITIS

It is generaly accepted that the fly *Hydrotaea irritans* is responsible for transmitting the bacteria responsible for summer mastitis. The correlations between aspects of the biology of the fly and the incidence of summer mastitis are considerable.

Prevention may consist of:

1. Taking zootechnical precautions with respect to sensitive animals in the risk period.

Examples of this include keeping the animals in the stall, as *H. irritans* is only found out of doors, or chosing pastures where summer mastitis is rare, *e.g.* on clay soils.

In recent years in the Netherlands, calves are pastured much later in the season, often towards the end of August and are soon (end September) re-stalled. Dry cows are also held indoors more, partially to prevent fat build up from a too large food availability. Heifers on the other hand, are generally pastured for the whole season from the 1st of May to the 1st of November, usually on distant pastures.

2. The use of preventive vaccination.

Up to now these have been relatively unsuccessful, probably due to complexity of the pathogen flora (Sol, 1983; Tolle *et al.*, 1985).

3. Protection of the teat duct opening/teat against flies.

This is a relatively old method. The results are generally disappointing as the particular treatments are usually applied incorrectly, too late and/or with insufficient frequency (Sol, 1984). However Danish reports (Klastrup, 1983) indicate positive results with "sealing" of teats. The treatment functions successfully if done at regular intervals.

4. Protection of the udder by using long acting antibiotics.

Good results have been obtained with long acting antibiotics even almost 40 years ago (Pearson, 1951). The treatment consisted of intramammary injection with 100,000 I.U. penicillin. This was carried out on 43 Irish farms where either the right or left quarters of 531 cows were treated at drying off. Injections were repeated 14 to 18 days later. Twenty-nine cases of summer mastitis in the 1062 untreated quarters whereas none occurred in the treated quarters.

Pearson reported that during the experiment 25 cases of mild infection were also discovered (18 in control and 7 in treated quarters). Bacteriological analysis revealed *S. dysgalactiae* (3), *S. agalactiae* (1), *S. aureus* (1), a non-haemolytic streptococ (1), *C. pyogenes* and 9 negative samples. All mild infections were healed completely with a single injection of 100,000 I.U. penicillin. Six of the summer mastitis infections could also be healed completely using the same treatment. According to Pearson this was due to immediate application on observing the clinical symptoms.

Pearson pointed out that it was remarkable how often cases of mild infection occur in dry cows. This may possibly be a predisposing factor for the occurrence of summer mastitis. These mild infections are less often seen when penicillin dry cow preparations are used. Pearson stated that Heave *et al.* (1950) also found many udder infections in the three weeks following drying up, which were presumably often present in the preceding lactation phase.

TABLE 1.   Comparison of summer mastitis in weeks after treatment of 2901 heifers with 250 mg cephalonium (Sol, 1982).

Weeks after treatment	1	2	3	4	5	6	7	8	>8 weeks	date unknown
Treated	—	—	—	1	1	3	6	6	17	
Control	3	9	1	5	6	15	7	9	21	16

According to Beimgraben (1983) Weight treated 841 heifers with two different long acting antibiotics in 1974 and 1975. The summer mastitis incidence in the treated and control groups was 0.7 and 12.5%, respectively. Beimgraben also obtained good results with long acting antibiotics. He recorded the first cases at least 44 days after treatment.

This is markedly longer than Sol's findings (see Table 1).

It is remarkable that S. *dysgalactiae* is so often found in summer mastitis in the U.K., but also in 1978 (Yeoman and Warren, 1984) often S. *uberis*. Edmonds and Welsch (1979), found that one treatment with a long acting antibiotic was insufficient to cover the dry period completely.

Treatment with long working antibiotics is too labour intensive and difficult for calves and heifers but is superior for dry cows and even preferable to ear-tags. It should, however, be re-applied 3 to 4 weeks after drying off.

5. Protecting the teat from *H. irritans*.

ODOURS: the use of strong smelling odours to repel flies is an old method which is now declining in use. One of the most well known is Stockholm tar. The results are doubtful (Sol, 1984) and its application is problematical, particularly with rather wild heifers. Another method is to introduce a billy-goat into the herd of heifers. This has been done by some farmers in the Netherlands but again with doubtful results.

INSECTICIDES: these are toxic and often repellant. Insecticides may be applied in several ways, *e.g.:*

a) *dust bags:* good results have been achieved with this method in the Netherlands (Kommerij, pers. com.) and in Germany (Beimgraben, 1983). The animals must walk under the dust bag frequently. For this reason the system is suitable for cows that are milked in the stall and can be forced to walk under the bag on leaving.

b) *sprays:* a large variety have long been available and used with success in preventing summer mastitis (Beimgraben, 1983). Their method of working and efficacy supports the hypothesis that flies play an important role in the occurrence of summer mastitis.

Sprays incorporating synthetic pyrethroids such as cypermethrin and permethrin have been used since the beginning of the 80's. They vary in effectiveness from 1 to 3 weeks (Titchener and Cochrane, 1980). The results obtained with sprays are good, given that they are applied sufficiently early, frequently and accurately (Bertels and Robijns, 1985; Tolle *et al.*, 1985).

However, results can often be disappointing (Sol, 1984). Yeoman and Warren (1984) also obtained poor results on dry cows which were regularly treated.

c) *the anti-summer mastitis box:* animals using this system are automatically sprayed during drinking. It is essential to check the system carefully and condition heifers expeditiously to the box. One disadvantage is the cost but the preventive working is good.

d) *pour-ons:* up to now the pour-ons used in the Netherlands contain the synthetic pyrethroid deltamethrin. They are effective from 4 to 6 weeks. They appear to be successful in reducing summer mastitis although this is difficult to say with certainty given the low incidence of the disease in the Netherlands over the last few years (Sol, 1984; Sol *et al.*, 1985).

Pour-ons and sprays are the most appropiate treatments for preventing summer mastitis in calves as they are usually given additional, concentrates daily and are easy to treat at this time. The same applies to milk cows where pour-ons are a potentially attractive method for controlling flies.

e) *ear-tags:* the incidence of summer mastitis is decreased when ear-tags are used (Table 2). The results were comparable to the effects obtained with long acting antibiotics (Table 3). Since 1982 ear-tags with different active compounds have become available. The efficacy appears to be high but the incidence of summer mastitis has been very low since 1982. Occasionally a severe outbreak has been observed despite the use of ear-tags. The infections reported in ear-tagged heifers in the summer are often caused by bacteria which are not typical for summer mastitis (Table 4 and Sol *et al.*, 1985). There also seems to be relatively more infections in the rear udders (Dommerholt, 1985), although this is not significant. In summer mastitis cases there is a significant tendency for infection of the fore udder (Dommerholt, 1985). This may indicate an exogenous influence in summer mastitis and an endogenous one in other udder infections during the summer.

TABLE 2.   Effect of ear-tags impregnated with Cypermethrin (Flectron®) on summer mastitis in 61 farms in Overijssel.

Year	1981	1982 (ear-tags)
Nr. of heifers	986	910
% summer mastitis	12.1%	0.9%
Average % of summer mastitis in Overijssel	3.4%	4.1%

TABLE 3.   Incidence of summer mastitis on 398 farms in Overijssel in 1982 (Sol, 1984)

	No. of heifers	% summer mastitis
Long acting antibiotics	2.202	1.5
Flectron® ear-tags	1.214	1.1
Other or no treatment	4.348	4.0

One marked difference between use of long acting antibiotics and ear-tags is the latency of the first summer mastitis cases after treatment. With long acting antibiotics no cases are seen until 3 to 4 weeks later whereas with ear-tags these may occur very soon after treatment (Fig. 1). As far as the latter are concerned, these are generally mild cases of infection that occasionally involve the typical *C. pyogenes* and/or anaerobe bacterial infection seen in summer mastitis but usually involve other bacteria. It is possible that a sub-clinical mastitis predisposes the development of a typical (see Sol *et al.*, section 1) summer mastitis. When long acting antibiotics are applied all (sub) clinical mastitis cases are inhibited for the first few weeks (Edmonds and Welsch, 1979; Sol and Vardy, 1982; Yeoman and Warren, 1984). After several weeks, as the long acting antibiotic becomes less effective the (sub) clinical mastitis reappears and, if flies are allowed access to the teat, typical summer mastitis cases occur (Sol *et al.*, 1985; Yeoman and Warren, 1984). Yeoman and Warren found that, using insecticides, a change occurred in the type of infection in that significantly far fewer *C. pyogenes* could be isolated. This change was not seen when antibiotics had been used.

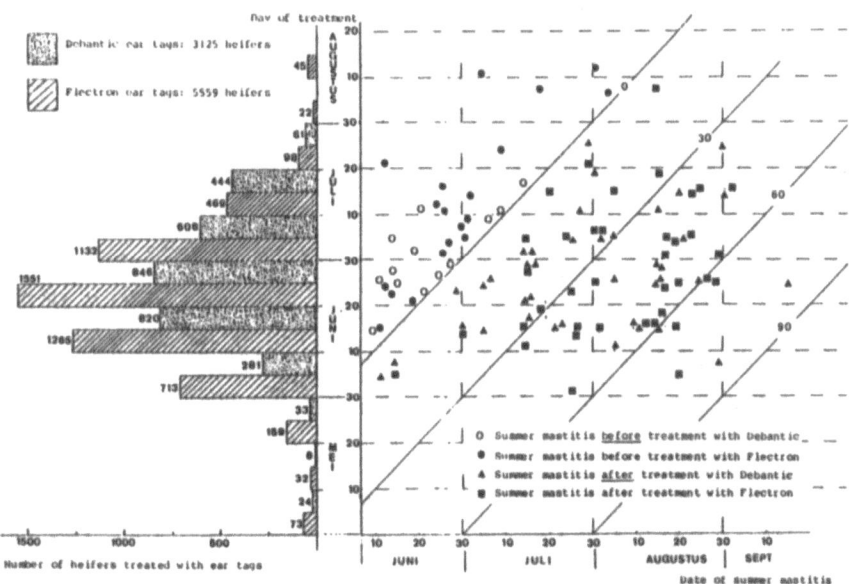

Fig. 1. Left: number of heifers treated with ear-tags at different times of the season.
Right: time of occurrence of the individual summer mastitis cases (abscissa) in relation to date of insertion of ear-tags (ordinate).

Ear-tags should not be inserted too close to the edge of the ear. It is also possible to utilize them as a neck band. If prevention of summer mastitis is the reason underlying the application of ear-tags then it is recommended to use two tags per animal (Taylor *et al.*, 1985).

Furthermore, it is essential to wash the hands thoroughly after insertion as several farmers have complained of headaches following treatment of animals.

Although resistance has not yet been recorded in the Netherlands it has become a problem in the U.S.A., particularly in areas where cattle flies have more than one cycle annually. To prevent the build up of resistance it is recommended to remove ear-tags when animals are brought into the stall at the end of the season.

The efficacy of ear-tags varies between farms. Large variation may also be present even between the fly populations on neighbouring meadows having essentially the same biotope. Whether or not this variation is constant between years has not yet been verified in the Netherlands.

In 1985, efficacy tests were carried out with ear-tags containing flucythrinate (Annual report of the Overijssel Animal Health Service, 1986). The results are presented in Table 5. It should be noted that the fly pressure was rather low in 1985 and no *Musca autumnalis* is found in the area.

TABLE 4.   Findings in 10 cases of udder infections occurring in the summers of 1984 and 1985 in ear-tagged heifers which calved later on.

Findings	Bacteriological category I and II	Bacteriological category III
No. of heifers	2	8
1 tag/heifer	1	1
2 tags/heifer	1	7
Systemic illness	2	0
Quarter: fore	1	4
Quarter: hard & swollen	2	0
Quarter: soft & swollen	0	8
Complete cure of udder tissue after treatment	0	8
Same bacteria still found 5 days later	2	0
Bacteriologically sterile 5 days later	0	5
Yellow secretion	2	8
Thick secretion	2	2
Thin secretion	0	6
Typical odour	0	0
Damaged teat opening	0	0

Category I & II = secretion contained *C. pyogenes* and/or obligate anaerobe bacteria.
Category III = absence of *C. pyogenes* and obligate anaerobe bacteria.

The same ear-tags have also been tested by Liebisch (1985) and in Denmark (Annual Report of the Danish Pest Infestation Lab., 1985).

Flucythrinate ear-tags still had the capacity to release insecticide 5½ months after insertion. Their efficacy against *H. irritans* was equally good in the 3rd and 4th month after application.

TABLE 5. Reduction of flies after applying flucythrinate containing, PVC ear-tags in 17 herds. The number of control herds was 12. Ear-tags were inserted from April 11 to May 15th.

Fly species	% Reduction	Significance
Hydrotaea irritans (Fallen)	64.1	p < 0.01
Hydrotaea albipuncta (Zetterstedt)	36.2	n.s.
Haematobia irritans (Linnaeus)	95.7	p < 0.001
Stomoxys calcitrans (Linnaeus)	61.5	p < 0.01
Haematobosca stimulans (Meigen)	38.4	p < 0.05
Tabanidae	41.2	n.s.

n.s. = not significant.

In the Netherlands, ear-tags are normally inserted in the beginning of May when animals are pastured. It is difficult to ascertain whether their efficacy is still sufficient to prevent summer mastitis in August. The reason for this is that the incidence of summer mastitis has been too low in the past few years, even on farms where no prevention methods are applied. Approximately 200 – 250,000 heifers are treated with ear-tags annually in the Netherlands with one of the 8 different ear-tags now available on the market. There appears to be very little difference between the efficacy of the different ear-tags.

PREVENTION IN HEIFERS CLOSE TO CALVING

Mastitis in this catagory of animals is often seen in almost all farms in the Netherlands. It usually involves only one animal but occasionally, particularly in winter, outbreaks involving many animals occur within a short period of time. Therapy is usually successfull. Prevention consists of twice daily teat dipping from one week prior to calving. Good results are also obtained by intramammary injection of Orbenin L.A. (Beecham) in each quarter the week before calving.

THE PREVENTION OF WINTER–C. PYOGENES MASTITIS

The so called "Winter-*C. pyogenes* mastitis" is found in both non-lactating and lactating animals in the Netherlands and is almost always attributable to teat injuries. The udder is generally lost for milk production. Prevention consists of improvement of laying facilities, selective breeding for more suitable teat and udder quality and good hoof care.

THERAPY OF SUMMER MASTITIS

Even if therapy is carried out, the quarter is generally lost as far as milk production is concerned in cases of summer mastitis. The best results that have been obtained so far are those of Heidrich and Fiebiger (1964, 1965). The therapy was carried out on 52 dry and lactating cows in which bacteriological examination confirmed the presence of a C. pyogenes infection. Therapy consisted of intramammary treatment with proteolytic enzymes (fibrolease and desoxy-ribonuclease) and antibiotics plus, in severe cases, intramuscular or intravenous injection of antibiotics. The udder tissues of 48% of the animals recovered completely and 27% partially. The quarter was completely lost in only 25% of the cases. Complete recovery could also be obtained with 4-6 week old infections in 35% of the quarters.

Saes (1971) used 20 cc intramammary injection of dimethylsulphoxide to which the proteolytic enzyme trypsin was added to treat 30 milk cows in which a C. pyogenes mastitis had been confirmed. Occasionally, additional treatment with intramuscular injection of antibiotic was carried out. Complete recovery was found only in 3 cases.

Buscher (1975) made use of the foam injection Ubrocelan® (Boehringer) with 63 summer mastitis heifers. Injection was carried out every 24 hrs and quarters were stripped frequently during the last half of the inter-injection period. Complete functional recovery of the udder tissue was found in 29 of the 63 animals.

Therapy trials were carried out in the Netherlands on 29 and 19 acute mastitis cases in pastured animals in 1984 and 1985, respectively. The animals consisted of 40 heifers, 5 calves and 3 dry cows. Veterinarians were requested to apply a standard therapy and collect samples anaerobically for bacteriological investigation. Records were kept of the clinical symptoms. The standard therapy in 1984 consisted of an intramuscular injection of 20% Spiramycin (Suanovil 20®, Rhone Poulenc) on the first and third day (Sol et al., 1985). On day 1 an intramammary treatment with an injector containing a spiromycine combination (Mammivert®, Rhone Poulenc) was also applied. The farmer was requested to keep the infected animals indoors for 5 days, to strip the secretion manually at regular intervals in the daytime and to apply a Mammivert injector each evening. A second secretion sample was taken on the 5th day. The same procedure was followed in 1985 but the standard therapy consisted of an intramuscular injection of 6 million IU Na-pen G and 10 million IU procain benzyl penicillin on the first day. An intramammary treatment with an injector containing 200 mg cloxalline and 75 mg ampiciline (Ampiclox®, Beecham) was applied on the first 5 consecutive evenings.

The results of the treatment are given in Table 6 for 24 heifers only.

Table 6 reveals that in the group where the udder is hard and swollen bacteria belonging to category III were found only once. This involved a staphylococcus infection and was the only udder in this group which healed completely. On the other hand, in the soft, swollen udder group, only one udder did not heal completely. In this case, a *S. uberis* infection was involved. Very little difference was found between the two treatments except that there appears to be a slight tendency that spiromycin has better effect if the infection belongs to category III.

The typical summer mastitis odour (Cornelisse *et al.*, 1970) appears to be a good diagnostic criterium. This was recorded 8 times in the total material for 1984 and 1985 and was always accompanied by a hard, swollen udder. However, *P. indolicus*, which is considered to be responsible for the odour, was only found in 2 of these 8 cases. Complete destruction of function was apparent in all 8 cases, the animals were usually very sick (7 cases) and all fell into category I or II. The colour of the secretion was yellow (7 cases) and thick (5 cases). The fore quarter was infected in 6 of the 8 cases. In none of these 8 cases had preventive measures been taken.

TABLE 6. Findings in 24 cases of udder infections occurring in the summers of 1984 and 1985 in 1 — 2 year old, pastured heifers which calved later on.

Characteristic	Individuals with hard, swollen udder		Individuals with soft, swollen udder	
	n	%	n	%
Number	11		13	
Systemic illness	10	91	1	8
Fore quarter	7	64	5	38
Damaged teat opening	2	18	1	8
Yellow secretion	9	82	12	92
White secretion	1	9	1	8
Red-brown secretion	1	9	0	
Thick secretion	6	54	3	23
Thin secretion	4	36	10	77
Lympy secretion	1	9	0	
Typical odour	3	27	0	
Ear-tagged	2	18	8	62
Complete cure of the udder tissue	1	9	12	92
Bacteria belonging to categories I & II*	10	91	0	
Bacteria belonging to category II**	1	9	13	100
Same bacteria found 5 days after treatment	8	73	1	8
Sterile 5 days after treatment	1	9	8	62

* Categories I & II contained *C. pyogenes* and/or obligate anaerobe bacteria.
**Category III contained other bacteria than in categories I and II.

The clinical aspects of the udder and the general condition of the heifer are the most important indicators for the prognosis. When the heifer has a systemic illness and/or the secretion has a distinct odour and/or the udder is hard and swollen (independent of the causative bacteria) the quarter will be usually lost, irrespective of therapy (Table 6).

When the udder is soft, oedematose and swollen, the prognosis is usually good. Farmers generally refer to these cases as being summer mastitis infections which are discovered very early. This is almost always incorrect as bacteriological investigation usually reveals species which are atypical for summer mastitis, such as S. uberis and other streptococci and staphylococci.

Application of a therapy is important in preventing the animal from becoming or remaining sick. In all cases where therapy was applied the animals become clinically healthy although, in most cases, the udder tissue is no longer functional.

It is necessary to bring the sick animal into the stall for efficient therapy. This also ensures that a source of the infection is removed from the pasture. Excision or incision of the teat is also possible. If the teat has been removed it is, however, essential not to replace these animals in the pasture as secretion containing C. pyogenes can continue to leak from the udder thus causing a large infection source.

It is necessary to inspect the remainder of the herd thoroughly as in 35% of the cases a new summer mastitis case will either occur directly or within a few days of the first case (Sol, 1983).

The value of a second bacteriological inspection on the 5th day only gives useful information in cases of category I and II infections.

If the teat remains swollen for several weeks and the sick quarter contains hard lumps then the prognosis is usually poor.

Diagnosis and prognosis is more difficult in cows. According to Weitz (1949) there is little difference between a summer mastitis udder infection and one caused by S. dysgalactiae as far as the clinical picture is concerned but the prognosis for a S. dysgalactiae is better. For this reason it is important to carry out bacteriological tests.

Cows often become seriously ill and can also die from summer mastitis infection. They often lie as they will not or can not stand. Infected heifers are readily identifiable as they usually stay isolated from the herd and walk rather stiffly. It is rare that heifers cannot stand. Calves are usually the least sick.

The best therapy is to treat the animal intramuscularly with antibiotics, strip the quarter frequently during the day and use an injector on the sick quarter in the evening. The therapy must be continued for at least 5 days.

ACKNOWLEDGEMENTS

We would like to thank the National Animal Health Committee, the Hague and the Central Veterinary Institute for their support of the summer mastitis project.

PREVENTION OF SUMMER MASTITIS BY FLY CONTROL:
A FIELD TRIAL WITH DELTAMETHRIN AS POUR—ON

G. Bertels

Verbond voor dierziektenbestrijding van Limburg,
Opsporingscentrum, Wetserstraat 14,
B 3820 — Alken, Belgium.

ABSTRACT

In 1983 a field trial for the prevention of summer mastitis was carried out using 2% deltamethrin as a pour on (Sputop-S[®]; Coopers). Treatment started in early June and was repeated after 6—9 weeks. In the 572 untreated controls 2.4% summer mastitis was diagnosed whereas in the 587 animals in the deltamethrin group the incidence was 0.2% (p = 0.006). The number of *Lyperosia irritans* increased steadily from 6 weeks after deltamethrin treatment and fly killing activity disappeared completely after 9 weeks. A cost/-benefit analysis per animal gave a profit of 7.7 E.C.U. in milk types and 2.8 E.C.U. in mixed types. This estimate was based on the very low incidence of 2.4% summer mastitis in 1983.

INTRODUCTION

A 4 year investigation was conducted into the incidence of summer mastitis in calves and heifers and a survey made of preventative methods. In the first year we examined the relative incidence of summer mastitis in different areas. Following this, we tested some new fly killing products on animals to ascertain their efficacy in reducing the number of *Hydrotaea irritans*, the suspected transmitter of summer mastitis. Tests were made on permethrin (Stomoxin EC[®]; Cooper) applied in an aqueous spray solution every 2 weeks, cypermethrin in ear-tags (Flectron[®]; Shell) 2 per animal. The results are given in Table 1. The two above mentioned methods gave a significant reduction of summer mastitis compared to the controls. In 1983 we tested the new synthetic pyrethroid, deltamethrin applied as a pour on (Sputop-S[®]; Coopers).

MATERIALS, METHODS AND RESULTS

Both control and treated herds were pastured on the sandy soil, wooded area of Limbourg in Belgium. These consisted mainly of black- and red and white heifers and calves of milk and mixed type cattle (see Bertels, Section 6).

Ten ml. of a 2% W/V deltamethrin suspension was applied on the back, paying particular attention to treating the anterior part of this region in order to avoid the suspension being wiped off by the tail before absorption. Five hundred and eighty-six animals were treated in this way about the 15th of June. Two hundred and ninety-two of these animals were re-treated after 6 weeks and the remaining 295 animals after a 9 week interval. The results for all 587 treated animals and the 572 untreated controls are given in Table 2.

TABLE 1. The results of different preventive treatments on the incidence of summer mastitis. N = number of animals; C = number of summer mastitis cases; % = percentage of summer mastitis cases
(data from Bertels and Robijns, 1983, 1985)

	1980			1981			1982			1983		
	N	C	%	N	C	%	N	C	%	N	C	%
Untreated	693	140	20.0	835	69	8.0	461	27	6.0	572	14	2.4
Permethrin sprayed				250	3	1.2**	274	6	2.0*			
Cypermethrin ear-tags							263	2	0.8**			
Deltamethrin pour on										587	1	0.2**

* = p < 0.05, ** = p < 0.001.

TABLE 2. Mean number of flies found on different areas of the body 5 and 9 weeks after treatment with Sputop-S® and just prior to the second treatment (6 weeks).
T = treated group; C = control group
(data from Bertels and Robijns, 1983, 1985)

	5 weeks		6 weeks		9 weeks	
	T	C	T	C	T	C
Back	0	> 100	8	> 100	> 100	> 100
Udder and legs	1	5	1	33	4	5
Head	40	30	8	25	6	15

DISCUSSION

As was expected on the basis of previous trials, the treatment gave a very good reduction of *Lyperosia irritans*. The number of these flies increased steadily from 6 weeks after deltamethrin application and fly killing activity had completely disappeared after 9 weeks. Reduction of other fly species was less, particularly on the head. We may therefore state that the maximum activity is a period of 6 weeks. Thus, in order to cover the fly season in Belgium we need a minimum of 2 treatments.

It is remarkable that summer mastitis incidence steadily decreased over the 4 years of the study. The same figures are also found in the Netherlands (Sol, 1983; Franken, 1983). Although the exact figures are not yet available for 1986 we had an impression that again a strong decrease occurred.

A cost/benefit analysis was attempted to determine the profit that might be expected from prevention with deltamethrin treatment. We took the loss per animal due to summer mastitis in milk types to be 444 E.C.U. and that of mixed types to be 222 E.C.U. Taking

100 heifers as a base line, the costs and benefits of deltamethrin treatment are set out in Table 3. The comparable data for 1 and 2 ear-tags are also included to give a relative measure. As far as the latter are concerned, we assumed that the relative incidences between control and treated groups were equivalent to those of the deltamethrin treatment (see Table 1) and moreover, earlier results indicated that no differences were present between 1 and 2 ear-tags under our conditions.

TABLE 3.   Gain in E.C.U. per 100 animals with different preventive treatments.
D = deltamethrin treatment; 1 ET and 2 ET = 1 and 2 ear-tags respectively.

| Cost | milk type (444 E.C.U./animal) | | | mixed type (222 E.C.U./animal) | | |
	D	1ET	2ET	D	1ET	2ET
Controls (2,4% s.m.)	1,065	1,065	1,065	533	533	533
Treated (0.2% s.m.)	89	89	89	44	44	44
Cost of treatment	204	444	888	204	444	888
Gain	772	532	88	285	45	- 399

The overall profit per animal if deltamethrin treatment is applied in a 2.4% summer mastitis year comes to 7.7 E.C.U. for milk types and 2.8 E.C.U. for mixed types.

THE ABILITY OF INSECTICIDAL EAR—TAGS, COLLARS, AND POUR—ONS TO CONTROL FLIES (DIPTERA: MUSCIDAE) AND TO PREVENT SUMMER MASTITIS IN HEIFERS

J.B. Jespersen and K.M. Vagn—Jensen

Danish Pest Infestation Laboratory,
Ministry of Agriculture,
Skovbrynet 14, DK—2800 Lyngby, Denmark.

ABSTRACT

Various plastic ear-tags, collars, and pour-ons containing pyrethroids and/or organo-phosphate were tested from 1983 to 1986 for their ability to control flies on pasturing heifers in Denmark. Some of the ear-tags were also assessed for the prevention of summer mastitis in heifers.

Double tagging of heifers in a five-month grazing period with 8.5% cypermethrin ear-tags gave complete control of the horn fly *Haematobia irritans* (100%) and was effective for control of *Haematobia stimulans* (93%), the sweat flies *Morellia* spp. (91%) and the head fly *Hydrotaea irritans* (67%). In the udder region the reduction of the head fly was 53%. Double tagging of heifers about 1 July with 8.5% cypermethrin ear-tags gave the following reductions for a three-month period: *Heamatobia irritans* (100%), *Haematobia stimulans* (91%), *Morellia* spp. (67%), *Hydrotaea irritans* (56%), and *Hydrotaea irritans* (udder) (35%).

A statistically significant reduction of 88% in the frequency of summer mastitis was obtained when two ear-tags were used on each of 685 heifers and compared with 798 untagged control heifers. The heifers were tagged about 1 July, just before outbreak of summer mastitis normally takes place in Denmark.

The efficacy of cypermethrin ear-tags is compared with the efficacy of other ear-tags, pour-ons, and collars, and different methods for fly control and disease prevention are discussed.

INTRODUCTION

Many sucking and biting diptera visit pasturing cattle to feed. In Denmark the most common biting Stomoxyinae on pasturing cattle are the horn fly, *Haematobia irritans* (L.) and *Haematobia stimulans* (Mg.), while the stable fly *Stomoxys calcitrans* (L.) is only seen on cattle grazing very close to a cowshed. The most common sucking fly is the head fly *Hydrotaea irritans* (Fall.), but *Morellia hortorum* (Fall.), *M. simplex* (Loew.), *Hydrotaea albipuncta* (Zett.), and *H. meteorica* (L.) are also quite common. *Musca autumnalis* De Geer is less frequent. The fauna of Diptera attacking pasturing cattle in Denmark is described in more detail by Petersen (1924), Ussing (1925), Thomsen (1938), Hammer (1941), Bahr (1955), Nielsen (1971), Nielsen and Christensen (1975), Nielsen et al., (1971, 1972), Jespersen (1981), Nielsen et al (1986), while the spatial distribution of various species of Diptera over the bodies of heifers is described by Jespersen et al. (1986).

In Denmark the main objective for controlling flies on pasturing cattle is a possible reduction in the frequency of the fly-transmitted disease, summer mastitis, an acute destructive polybacterial infection of the udder in non-lactating cattle. *Hydrotaea irritans* is assumed to be the main transmitter of this disease (Tarry *et al.*, 1978; Sorensen, 1974; Hillerton *et al.*, 1983). *Moraxella bovis*, the pathogen of Keratoconjunctivitis, may be transmitted by several fly species, *i.e. Musca autumnalis* (Brown and Adkins, 1972), *Hydrotaea irritans* and *Morellia* species, which are active in the eye region of the cattle. The biting and sucking Diptera species are irritant to grazing cattle, but they are not considered to cause any significant weight or milk loss in Denmark (Jespersen, 1984), although they may cause some unrest.

One of the main reasons for fly control on pasturing cattle in many southern countries and in the USA is the presence of the horn fly, *Haematobia irritans*, which causes weight and milk loss in cattle. Various insecticides formulated as sprays, ear-tags, collars, dusts, and pour-ons have been evaluated for control of this fly species. Excellent control of the horn fly can be achieved by all these methods, but resistance in the fly is now widespread and increasing (Sheppard, 1984; Byford *et al.*, 1985; Schmidt *et al.*, 1985; Sparks *et al.*, 1985). Control of the non-biting, sucking Diptera is generally more difficult, but may be important as several of these flies may transmit diseases among cattle, *e.g.* summer mastitis by *Hydrotaea irritans*, pink eye by *Musca autumnalis* and *Hydrotaea irritans*, and Parafilariosis by *Musca autumnalis* (Bech-Nielsen *et al.*, 1982).

MATERIALS AND METHODS

The most common breed of cattle in Denmark is the Holstein-Friesian, or Black and White Dairy Cattle, and as this race has the highest frequency of summer mastitis, it was decided to use only heifers belonging to this race in the study. All the treated heifers were provided with two 10 gram 8.5% w/w cypermethrin ear-tags each using the All-flex tagging system. Treated and control herds of heifers were always separated with at least a double fencing to prevent cross-contamination. They grazed in comparable pastures with respect to topography and insect activity.

Control of insect activity

This investigation was made in 1985 in four localities. In two localities, at Varde and at Aalestrup, the ear-tags were applied on 15 April while they were applied on 2 July in St. Vildmose and on 9 July in Ll. Vildmose. Each herd consisted of at least 20 heifers (mainly in calf) and was compared to a similar control group grazing nearby with respect to insect activity. The number of flies on 20 heifers in both groups was counted weekly from turn out in late May until early October, preferably on windless, hot days with a high humidity, and between 10 *a.m.* and 4 *p.m.* Fly counts were made within one hour in each locality, and only finished if the weather conditions remained constant. Separate counts were made on six regions on one side of the heifer's body, *i.e.* head, back, side, belly, udder, and legs. Within each region the number of flies belonging to one of the test species, *Haematobia irritans, Haematobia stimulans, Hydrotaea irritans*, and *Morellia* spp., was recorded. Usually counts were made by direct observation, but from time to time binoculars were used in order not to disturb the herd. To minimize the influence on the recordings of heterogeneous fly distribution caused by sunlight or breeze, and by individual differences among heifers, the heifers were selected at random as the observer walked around or through the herd. Identification of the test species in the field was possible due to the study of flies on pasturing heifers made during the previous years. From time to time flies were netted and identified in the laboratory.

The percentage reduction of flies was calculated as:

$$((C-T)/C) \times 100$$

where C is the mean number of flies on the control heifers, and T is the mean number of flies on the tagged heifers. A probit analysis revealed that the data from the fly observations were approximately normally distributed when transformed to $(\ln(C+1)-\ln(T+1))$. Therefore the paired t-test (used for paired observations) was used with the transformed data to test if the percentage reduction was significant at a 5% level.

Control of summer mastitis

In four localities in Jutland, at Varde, Aalestrup, Moldrup, and Ll. Vildmose, a total of 697 heifers and dry cows were double-tagged with cypermethrin ear-tags from 20 June and until 10 July. All heifers were registered with respect to breed, locality, tagging date, grazing period, status of pregnancy (calf, in calf, not in calf), date of observation of summer mastitis, lost ear-tags, and a description of the pasture. Registration of summer mastitis was based on reports from the farmers and the local veterinarians. In this investigation, summer mastitis was defined as an observed acute inflammation of the udder in the heifer during the grazing period until the date of calving.

Each herd of tagged heifers was compared with a similar control group consisting of untreated heifers grazing in the same area, altogether 804 heifers and dry cows. A total of 46 farmers with treated and control heifers took part in the trail. The data were analysed statistically using a chi-square test when all the data were gathered.

RESULTS

Fly counts were initiated in Aalestrup and Varde in late May at turn out and at the beginning of July in St. Vildmose and Ll. Vildmose, and continued until the beginning of October in all localities. The four test species were present in all localities, and constituted more than 95% of the total number of insects. *Hydrotaea irritans* was present from late June until mid-September, with the highest numbers from mid-July to mid-August. The two biting flies, *Haematobia stimulans* and *Haematobia irritans* were present during the whole trial period in all localities, with *Haematobia irritans* most common during late June, July and August and *Haematobia stimulans* most common in the autumn. The *Morellia* species were sporadic in all localities, and most common in July-August. The fly activity was, in general, highest in Aalestrup, especially with respect to the horn fly. The number of the head fly *Hydrotaea irritans* was uniform in all localities except for Li. Vildmose, where there were only half as many head flies per heifer as in the other localities.

The percentage reduction of the fly test species is given in Table 1 for each of the four localities. For *Hydrotaea irritans* the percentage reduction is also given for the udder region in view of the importance of this fly as a transmitter of summer mastitis. *Hydrotaea irritans* was only partly controlled. The control of fly numbers in the udder region was not as efficient as for the whole heifer. In general, the control was surprisingly better for heifers tagged at turn out than for cattle tagged in July. The same applied to the *Morellia* species, which were reduced by a mean of 91% if the heifers were tagged in early spring, but by 67% if they were tagged at the beginning of July. The biting horn fly, *Haematobia irritans* was totally controlled in all localities, while *Haematobia stimulans* was reduced in number by more than 90%. The control of these two biting flies was independent of the length of the trial period (3 or 5 months).

TABLE 1. **Percentage reduction of fly test species for heifers tagged before turn out (Aalestrup and Varde) and for heifers tagged just before outbreak of summer mastitis (St. Vildmose and Ll. Vildmose).**

Tagging date	Locality	*Hydrotaea irritans* total	udder	*Haematobia irritans*	*Heamatobia stimulans*	*Morellia* spp.
15 April	Aalestrup	74*	58	100*	96*	92*
15 April	Varde	59*	48*	100*	89*	93*
15 April	Combined	67*	53*	100*	93*	91*
2 July	St. Vildmose	59*	38	100*	89*	62
9 July	Ll. Vildmose	47	29	99*	92*	62
2, 9 July	Combined	56*	35	100*	91*	67*

* $p < 0.05$.

The paddocks where the tagged and the control heifers were grazing showed only minor differences in topography and habitat and it was concluded that they were comparable with respect to fly populations and potential for summer mastitis. The number of farms and cattle and the number and percentage of summer mastitis cases are given for each locality in Table 2. The number of control and tagged cattle and cases of summer mastitis are given for calves, virgin heifers, heifers in calf, and dry cows in Table 3. In all four localities and in each subgroup of heifers, some or complete control of summer mastitis was obtained. Only one case of summer mastitis was seen in the tagged group of cattle, whereas ten cases were found in the control group. Although the total number of cases was very low the results showed an overall statistically significant (5 per cent level) control of summer mastitis of 88%.

TABLE 2. The numbers of farms, tagged and control cattle and the incidence of summer mastitis for the four trial localities.

Locality with number of farms in brackets	No. of cattle	Tagged cattle		No. of cattle	Control cattle	
		Summer mastitis			Summer mastitis	
		No.	%		No.	%
Aalestrup (3)	52	0	0	85	1	1.2
Moldrup (2)	65	0	0	60	1	1.7
Ll. Vildmose (18)	159	0	0	204	3	1.5
Varde (23)	421	1	0.2	455	5	1.1
Total without dry cows	685	1	0.1	798	10	1.3

TABLE 3. The numbers of control and tagged cattle and the number and percentage reduction of summer mastitis in each subgroup.

Subgroup	Tagged heifers		Control heifers		Percentage reduction
	Total	Infected	Total	Infected	
Calf up to one year	51	0	131	1	100
Heifers not in calf	305	1	352	3	62
Heifers in calf	329	0	315	6	100
Dry cows	12	0	6	0	—
Total (calves and heifers)	685	1	798	10	88

CONCLUSIONS AND DISCUSSION

The present study showed a significant control of fly infestation on pastured cattle double tagged with 8.5% cypermethrin ear-tags for more than five months. The biting horn fly, *Haematobia irritans* was easily and totally controlled. The level of control achieved for the other test fly species was, presented as means for a grazing period in four different localities: *Haematobia stimulans* 89—96%, *Hydrotaea irritans* 47—74%, *Hydrotaea irritans* (udder) 29—58%, and *Morellia* spp. 62—93%. In 1984 a similar trial was conducted in Denmark (Jespersen and Vagn—Jensen, 1985). The results obtained for animals tagged around 1 July were very similar to the present ones, except for *Hydrotaea irritans* where the level of control was as high as 87% for the whole animal, and 83% in the udder region (means for two localities). In a five-month-trial in 1984, the results obtained were influenced very heavily by massive attacks of blackflies (Simuliidae). The activity of the blackflies, causing bleeding and wounds, presumably influenced the efficacy of the ear-tags, and no control of the sucking flies *Hydrotaea irritans* and *Morellia* spp. was seen.

Very similar results to those presented in Table 1 and in the three-month-trial in 1984 have been obtained in the UK with two cypermethrin ear-tags (Hillerton *et al.*, 1985; Wright *et al.*, 1984). However, if one ear-tag was used per individual no control of *Hydrotaea irritans* was obtained in the udder region, and the total fly control was slightly poorer, 90% in comparison to 99% (Hillerton *et al.*, 1985). In northern Germany in 1985, Liebisch found cypermethrin to be effective at a high level for five months; moreover, a control of about 95% was obtained for *Hydrotaea irritans*. The same result was found in Belgium in 1985 by Pecheur, who reported a 90% reduction in the numbers of *Hydrotaea irritans*.

Trials were conducted from 1984—85 in Denmark to evaluate the ability of several pyrethroids, organophosphates or combinations, formulated as ear-tags, collars or pour-ons, to control flies on pasturing cattle. Besides cypermethrin, four other pyrethroids (fenfluthrin, fluvalinate, fenvalerate, and flucythrinate), two organophosphates (propetamphos and tetrachlorinphos) and one combination (fenvalerate/propetamphos) all incorporated in ear-tags, have been shown to control flies on pasturing cattle, at least, for a three-month-period, (Jespersen, 1984; Jespersen and Vagn—Jensen, 1985, 1986). Liebisch (1985), demonstrated that permethrin ear-tags were able to control flies on pasturing cattle in northern Germany. In Denmark, a collar containing fluvalinate and propetamphos was effective for at least a three-month-period against *Hydrotaea irritans, Haematobia irritans, Haematobia stimulans*, and *Morellia* spp., while monthly treatment of pastured cattle on the back with 10 or 20 ml cyfluthrin resulted in control of the the same fly species at the same level as obtained with the ear-tags (Jespersen, 1984; Jespersen and Vagn—Jensen, 1985, 1986).

Control of flies on pasturing cattle might result in a reduction of disease incidence of fly transmitted diseases. The present investigation showed a reduction of summer mastitis incidence by 88% with two cypermethrin ear-tags per heifer applied around 1 July. Similar results were obtained in 1983—85 with fenvalerate (67%), fluvalinate (71%), flucythrinate (57%), and propetamphos (53%) ear-tags in three-month-trials, but almost no control was obtained if the ear-tags were applied at turn out of the cattle in May (Jespersen, 1984; Jespersen and Vagn–Jensen, 1985, 1986). Bertels and Robijns (1983) reduced the incidence of summer mastitis by 97% with two cypermethrin ear-tags per heifer applied on or about 20 June in a trial in Belgium. In Germany, Hofmann (1985) reduced the incidence of summer mastitis to 0.5% of the tagged heifers compared to 13.0% in the control animals.

The feeding activity of the biting Diptera, *e.g. Haematobia irritans* and Simuliidae species results in bleeding wounds on the animals, and consequently the sucking Diptera *Hydrotaea irritans* and the *Morellia* spp. are more attracted to the cattle. The control of *Hydrotaea irritans* may therefore rely partly on the control of the biting flies. In fact, in a locality where many blackflies were feeding on the pasturing cattle no control of the sucking flies was obtained (Jespersen and Vagn–Jensen, 1985). Development of resistance in horn flies to the insecticides used for control of flies on cattle may therefore result in less control of *Hydrotaea irritans*, and consequently, in reduced or no control of summer mastitis. Until now, no resistance in *Haematobia irritans* has been observed in Denmark probably due to fewer generations of this fly than in the USA, and less widespread use of ear-tags. In the USA, resistance to pyrethroids in *Haematobia irritans* is common.

The benefit of ear-tags for the control of flies on cattle is that only one treatment is needed per summer. However, many farmers tend not to remove the ear-tags when bringing cattle in for the winter period, and this will increase the risk of rapid and widespread resistance in the populations of the houseflies *Musca domestica* on the farms. In Denmark, ear-tags have to be removed from cattle in winter time for this reason. The use of pour-ons might seem more laborous as at least monthly treatment of cattle is required, but in fact treatments are carried out very easily. With the pour-ons used on pastured cattle the same resistance problems will probably not appear in farm or field populations of flies.

RESULTS OF THE CONTROL OF FLIES AND SUMMER MASTITIS BY USING DIFFERENT PYRETHROIDS AND FORMS OF APPLICATION IN GERMANY

A. Liebisch

Institute of Parasitology,
Department of Veterinary Entomology,
Veterinary School Hannover,
Bunteweg 17, D — 3000 Hannover, F.R. Germany.

ABSTRACT

Summer mastitis in heifers is a widespread infection in Germany causing losses up to 14% in certain herds and areas. Since the introduction of pyrethroids into veterinary medicine, trials have been performed for control of flies and prevention of summer mastitis in grazing cattle. In controlled field trials involving hand spraying, the pyrethroids permethrin, cypermethrin, deltamethrin and cyfluthrin were used, followed by trials with ear tags containing permethrin, cypermethrin, cyhalothrin, fenvalerate and flucythrinate. Finally pour-ons were used containing deltamethrin, cypermethrin, cyfluthrin and cyhalothrin. The protection period for excellent fly control was 21 days after hand spraying, 4 — 5 months with the ear tags and 35 days with the pour-ons. After early spring treatment with ear tags, a much better control of flies resulted than with the summer treatment. In controlled field trials, summer mastitis in heifers could be reduced in treated animals to 2.4% compared with 12.5% infected heifers in the untreated herds.

INTRODUCTION

The relation between flies and summer mastitis in cattle was discussed even before the turn of the century in the German veterinary literature when Dieckerhoff (1878), Reimers (1888) and Nielsen (1908) described the so called "Holsteinische Euterseuche" in North Germany. Until recently the disease was believed to occur in the northern parts of Germany only but recent studies (Hofmann, 1985) indicate that the disease extends much more to the south of the country where a high disease incidence (13%) is seen. There were many efforts made to control summer mastitis by using insecticides against the vector flies in Germany. In the fifties, trials with DDT and BHC were performed by Götze (1951), Aehnelt (1955), Malze (1957) and Lindloff (1958). Almost 20 years later coumaphos (Asuntol) in dust bags gave good results in trials by Weight and Lindfeld (1976). Finally, the introduction of pyrethroids into veterinary medicine in Germany, starting with permethrin and cypermethrin in 1981/82, opened new ways and possiblities for control of flies and disease (Elger and Liebisch, 1982; Künast *et al.*, 1983; Liebisch 1983 a, 1983 b, 1984, 1985, 1986; Hofmann, 1985).

MATERIALS AND METHODS

Between 1981 and 1986 most of the trials were conducted in an area close to Hannover where the fly fauna composition and many other biological data on flies associated with cattle are known from previous studies (Liebisch and Elger, 1983; Elger, 1985). The area consisted of grassland with moor and woodland transversed by ditches. In this enzootic area of summer mastitis of heifers, the herds for trials were selected so that the type of pasture and the animals involved would permit comparable figures to be achieved. The herds were, however, sufficiently separated to prevent them from affecting one another. As a rule, there was at least one unoccupied pasture between 2 test herds. A total of 5.100 animals were included in the different trials.

The various species of flies and tabanids were established by catching the Diptera on the animals, and a special herd was kept for the purpose of catching the insects. These animals had become accustomed to the presence of research workers and catching procedures. Our field reports included the effect of the pyrethroids on the flies and tabanids visually recognisable in the field. The following species or genera could be distinguished at a distance of about 2 m:

Haematobia irritans, by far the most prevalent fly found on the back of the cattle, the bigger biting fly *Haematobia stimulans* and *Musca autumnalis*, the only musca variety in the pastures. *Hydrotaea* could only be distinguished as a genus, however *H. irritans* and *H. albipuncta* were the only prevalent species in the area. *Haematopota* spec. was the only tabanid present in large numbers and with a sufficient long period of activity (June to August). There were also large tabanids of the genus *Hybomitra, Chrysops* and *Tabanus*, though these were not included in the assessment because of their brief period of activity and their relatively small numbers. The various species of *Morellia*, present only in small numbers, and *Stomoxys calcitrans* also present in small numbers in pastures at some distance from the shed, were excluded because of their insignificance in the test area.

The species *Haematobia irritans* was used as an indicator species for the assessment of the duration of the action of a pyrethroid. This fly is known to be a stationary living ectoparasite in its imaginal stage. Therefore, the reappearence of this fly after treatment was considered as the end of any repellent or insecticidal effect. The intensity of fly infestation was assessed by means of visual counts of the above mentioned flies and tabanids on 10 animals. The count was taken once a week between 9 a.m. and 3 p.m. on standing animals. All of the resting or biting flies on the animals body and head were counted. No count was made when it was raining.

The area under study is well known for the enzootic occurrence of summer mastitis in heifers. Veterinarians and cattle breeders are very familiar with the disease. The rates of clinical cases in treated and untreated heifers were compared for establishing the data on summer mastitis. In treated heifers, the infection was confirmed by microbiological demonstration of *C. pyogenes*. In the untreated animals, the diagnosis was made according to the typical clinical symptoms such as swelling of the udder and the typical smell of the secretion. However, most of the cases were not laboratory confirmed. The figures demonstrated may therefore be considered slightly high, because some cases of mastitis having another cause may be included. There is, however, a general agreement that clinical and laboratory confirmed diagnosis in enzootic areas of summer mastitis do not differ by more than 20%.

RESULTS

Pyrethroids, application and results of fly control

The different pyrethroids and methods of application are listed in Table 1. For *hand spraying* the permethrin was used in a 20% formulation of 25:75 cis-trans ratio (Stomoxin MO) diluted to 1:200 in the amount of 500 ml per animal. All treatments resulted in a very good onset of action. After the first 15 minutes the animals were free from any kind of flies. Almost 100% control was achieved in biting flies for 14 days, and more than 90% for 21 days. In non-biting flies more than 80% control was found for 14 days. There was a good control in all types of flies for 21 days after hand spraying (Fig. 1).

TABLE 1. **The pyrethroids and the forms of application for control of flies in grazing cattle in Germany (1981 — 1986)**

PYRETHROID	SPRAY	EAR-TAG	POUR-ON
Cyhalothrin	—	+	+
Cyfluthrin	+	—	+
Cypermethrin	+	+	+
Deltamethrin	+	—	+
Fenvalerate	—	+	—
Flucythrinate	—	+	+
Permethrin	+	+	—

+ Trials performed in Germany, — No trials in Germany.

Four treatments were needed for good fly control during the entire grazing season (4 — 5 months). In spite of the availability of easier methods of application, hand spraying is the most reliable method.

Later on, trials were performed with hand spraying of deltamethrin, cypermethrin and cyfluthrin. The results of fly control, onset and duration of the action were similar to the results with permethrin. However in several cases the irritation of the mucous membrane of the nostrils and the eyes was so strong that the trails were discontinued.

176

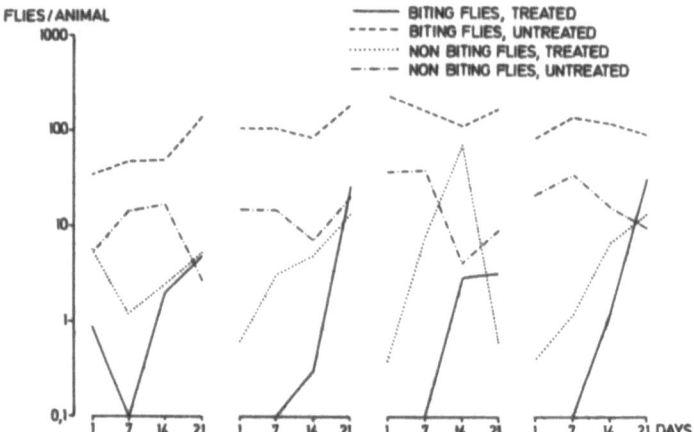

Fig. 1. The effect of hand spraying permethrin (500 mg a.i. animal) for control of flies in cattle.

To avoid the disadvantage of collecting animals on the pasture for spraying, a *self-application box for spraying* coupled to a self-drinking water pump was used to apply permethrin to the ventral surface and the udder region of the animals during drinking (Liebisch, 1983 b). During the 4 year use of this equipment (made in Holland) we observed a very effective and reliable action. The control of flies was almost 90%, and in a small herd of 16 very valuable heifers no case of summer mastitis occurred during the 4 years of study compared to 1 — 3 heifers/year infected with summer mastitis in the years before treatment.

Trials with the *pour-on technique* for control of flies in Germany were first performed with deltamethrin (Fig. 2). Later on, trials with cypermethrin, cyfluthrin and cyhalothrin were performed. For this reason, the results achieved with deltamethrin were used as a standard to compare the results obtained with the other pyrethroids. The big advantage of the pour-on application will not be further explained here. The method is the most preferable one in dairy cows but less practicable in heifers, in feed lots and on pastures. With all the pyrethroids used in our trials, almost 100% control of biting flies *(Haematobia irritans, H. stimulans)* and 90% control of non-biting flies *(Musca autumnalis, Hydrotaea* spec.) was achieved for 30 — 35 days after treatment (Fig. 2). There was a very small and statistically non-significant difference in the duration period (reappearance of *H. irritans* between day 30 and 35) with the different pyrethroids and formulations used.

After the second pour-on treatment the population development of biting flies in the area was completely interrupted. With all 4 pyrethroids studied, an excellent fly control was achieved with 3 — 4 treatments during the 5 month grazing season in Germany.

Nowadays the application of *insecticidal ear-tags* is the most practicable method for fly control in grazing heifers in Germany. The one to two year old cattle are usually seen by the owner "twice a year" during the grazing season, once at turning out in spring and once when brought back in fall. Therefore, long acting ear-tags are the method of first choice.

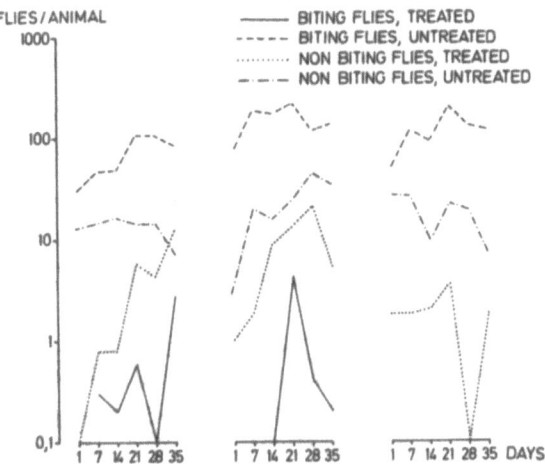

Fig. 2. Results of the control of flies in grazing cattle after application of deltamethrin as pour-on.

With the 5 types of pyrethroid ear-tags under study (Table 1) a 60 — 80% reduction of non-biting flies and a 90 — 100% reduction of biting flies was achieved. Differences in fly numbers seen on the cattle with different pyrethroid ear-tags were caused by the kind of fixation or the type of the plastic or rubber carrier rather than by the incorporated pyrethroid. Losses of ear-tags by broken "necks" and alteration in the ear-tag material were of greater influence on the fly numbers than the pyrethroids used. A representative figure of the action of insecticidal ear-tags on biting and non-biting flies is given in Figure 3. The total fly burden is shown here, biting and non-biting flies being counted together. The effective duration in fly control was during a 140 day period between May and October. The reduction in the fly numbers was more than 95% throughout the grazing period.

There is however, a clear difference between early and late tagging. After early treatment, the fly populations are not able to build up to the regular abundance. The early breeding activity of the overwintering adults (Musca autumnalis) or of the emerging females of the first spring generation (Hydrotaea and Haematobia spec.) is strongly disturbed by preventing the female flies from feeding on the animal protein (in the form of mucous or blood) which is needed for the development of their eggs. With early treatment there are even periods when no flies are found on the cattle. Later on in the year (during summer) the development of the fly populations is continuously disturbed, reaching numbers of less than 10 flies/animal compared to 200 flies/animal in untreated controls (Fig. 3).

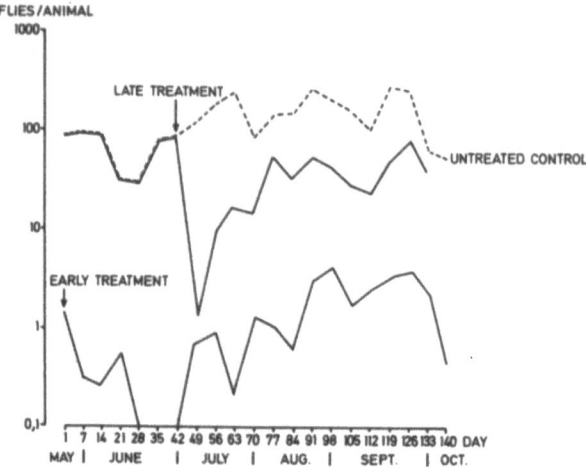

Fig. 3. The effect of pyrethroid ear-tags on the flies on grazing cattle after early and late tagging in the year.

Using late tagging however, the effect of treatment can be more impressive for the unexperienced observer because the abundance of flies has already reached fairly high numbers in June (a 100 or more) and tagging reduces the numbers of flies (mainly *Haematobia irritans*) in an impressive manner for the following weeks of high fly activity. This effect will last for the highly susceptible and stationary living *Haematobia irritans* over summer and fall. However, the action of treatment will be of limited effect on the further generations of emerging flies of the non-biting type (*Musca autumnalis, Hydrotaea* spec.) which will reach certain numbers during late summer and fall (Fig. 3).

In some parts of our trials we used *tag-tapes* containing 0.9 g cyhalothrin in 2 small ampules. With this method we also registered a very good result with a reduction of 100% in biting and 90% in non-biting flies. With the ear-tag-tapes a way has been found to combine the large plastic ear-tags which already exist in many farms with an impregnation of insecticide. The fixation of the tapes is a little more time consuming but the advantages are obvious.

Results in control of summer mastitis by control of flies

There is no doubt that effective control of flies does not implicitly and always mean an effective control of summer mastitis. There are many herds known in which cases of summer mastitis occurred despite the control of flies. However, larger scale trials confirm that control of flies considerably reduces the risk of infection in treated animals.

In our studies we selected herds of heifers known for high risk of infection, with summer mastitis occurring in the herds year after year. During the years 1982 — 1986 we treated 668 heifers in 26 herds with ear-tags containing permethrin, cypermethrin, cyhalothrin, fenvalerate and flucythrinate. Because these herds were included in trials for the investigation of the effectivity of different pyrethroids in ear-tags against flies, different pyrethroids in tags were used in subsequent years. The herds remained the same throughout the 4 years but the animals were changed after calving and the number differed slightly from year to year.

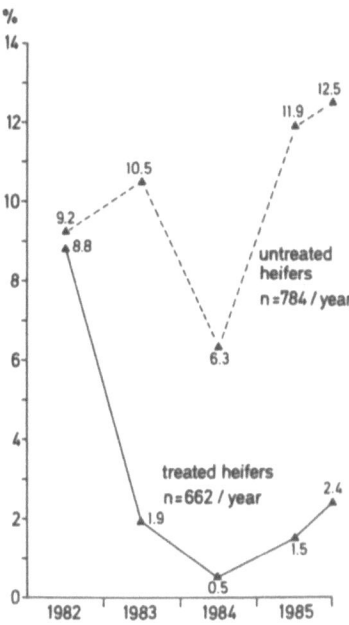

Fig. 4. Clinical cases of summer mastitis in heifers treated with insecticidial ear-tags (pyrethroids) and in untreated heifers in an enzootic area.

In the surroundings of the treated animals, 784 heifers in 31 herds were selected for use as untreated controls. Only herds with a known, high risk of summer mastitis were chosen. The main part of these herds remained the same during the study but 11 of the herds had to be replaced by other herds because the owners decided to treat the heifers against flies with pyrethroids which became available on the market.

During the trials, all cases of summer mastitis in heifers occurring on the pasture during the grazing season and in fall (late recognized) were reported. Starting with the tagging of 1 year old heifers in 1982 all 1 and 2 years old heifers were tagged in the following years. There was a significant decline in cases with summer mastitis in the herds with ear-tags compared to the untreated cattle. The number of cases in treated animals increased from 1984 until the winter of 1985/86. However, this rise was much less than the steep rise of clinical cases in untreated herds during the same time. There is no doubt of the value of fly control for controlling summer mastitis.

PREVENTION AND THERAPY OF SUMMER MASTITIS:
OBSERVATIONS OF FIELD OUTBREAKS IN THE UNITED KINGDOM

C.A. Watson

Ministry of Agriculture, Fisheries and Food,
Veterinary Investigation Centre, Langford,
Langford House, Bristol, U.K.

ABSTRACT

A large number of heifers were monitored over four years (1983-1986) in the south-west of England. The distribution and incidence of affected animals was observed as were the preventive measures employed and therapies applied. Disease was reported by veterinary surgeons and followed up with a questionnaire. The real incidence was difficult to assess but genuine changes were appreciable through contact with private veterinary surgeons. Incidence has been low and coincides with the introduction and use of insecticide impregnated ear-tags. However, many premises experienced severe outbreaks in 1986 despite their continued use. Farmers have frequently commented that insecticides used as a spray or pour-on are more effective than ear-tags at removing flies. Therapy is aimed at minimising deaths rather than in curing, with the animal being lost from the dairy. In January 1986, a herd of milking cows experienced an outbreak of mastitis bearing close similarities to summer mastitis, both bacteriologically and clinically. Although Mycoplasmas have been associated, their significance remains unknown. There was a total absence of flies.

OBSERVATIONS OF FIELD OUTBREAKS IN THE UNITED KINGDOM

The field outbreaks of summer mastitis observed were confined to the south-west of England and in particular the counties of Avon, Somerset, Dorset and Wiltshire.

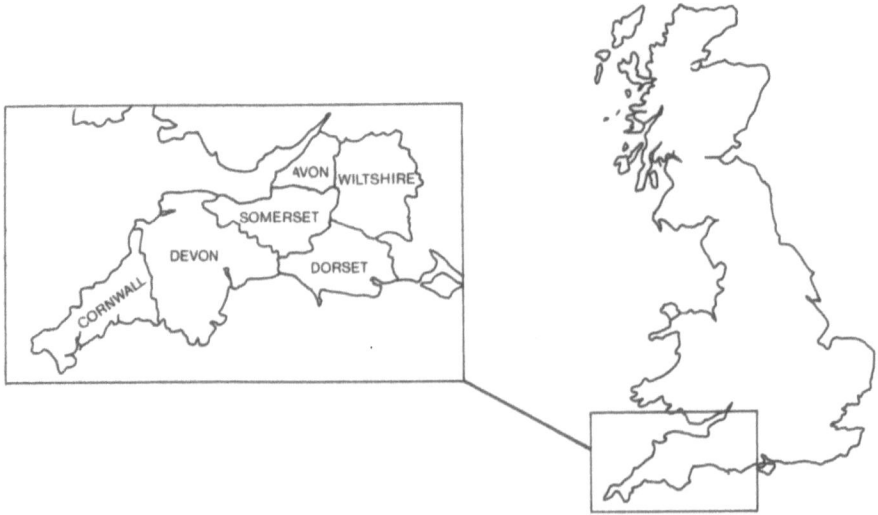

| County | Cattle Population x 10^3 | |
	Dairy	Beef
Avon	47	3.8
Somerset	114.5	8.6
Dorset	157.7	19.6
Wiltshire	92.9	11.3
	412.1*	43.8

*46,000 registered producers of milk.

Taking an estimate of 10 per cent replacement per annum, the heifer population is: 40,000 6 months — 18 months, 40,000 18 months — 30 months.

With the present trend towards autumn calving, then a high proportion of the older heifers would be in late pregnancy during July, August and September. As the clinical condition is readily recognised by the farmer, many cases are dealt with by him alone, whether this is treatment or culling. Accurate data on actual incidence is difficult to record. Estimates have been attempted (O'Rourke, MMB 1984) suggesting incidence within groups of susceptible animals as 0.6 — 1.9 per cent (O'Rouke et al., 1985). Incidence itself is highly unpredictable. In the same article, 1981 was a high incidence year, particularly amongst dry cows. This was confirmed in this area by the number of reports from veterinary surgeons in practice. In many cases outbreaks involved up to 50 per cent of groups of heifers together with dry cows. An intriguing feature was the appearance of clinical disease over a large area almost simultaneously between August 28 and 31, 1981.

As is experienced in other diseases such as Liver Fluke (Fascioliasis), the year following a high incidence was of low incidence. Was this a natural effect or the result of effective preventive measures being applied? The introduction of insecticide impregnated ear-tags (IIET) was slowly taken up in 1983 but by 1986 the practice is very common in both cows and all ages of young stock. Reports have been received throughout the south-west of England that summer mastitis has been very common, though later, this year. Many animals have been affected within groups at risk. In many if not most instances, IIET have been employed. Following up these outbreaks showed that woodlands were close by (frequently deciduous only) and that running water in the form of streams was also present. However in some significant cases tree or hedge cover and water were absent. The behaviour of the cattle suggested that the use of one ear-tag per animal controlled the nuisance flies well (Hillerton et al., in press; Wright et al., 1984). On one farm, 8/30 heifers were affected between the end of July and the end of September 1986. Ear-tags were applied at the beginning of July. Another group of heifers on the same farm, some two kilometers away, had no cases of summer mastitis. Sheep also graze in adjacent fields and there has been no history of sheep head fly either this year or in the past. Generally unfavourable comments have been received about IIET fly control and summer mastitis (Hillerton *et al.*, 1982). Insecticides in the form of pour-on and sprays are felt to be more effective though less convenient (Bramley *et al.*, 1985).

A variety of treatments exist perhaps reflecting the complexity of this condition and also the generally poor response (Yeoman and Warren, 1984). This year, however, several reports have commented upon very favourable results using parenteral Erythromycin with and without non-steroidal anti-inflammatory drugs. Drainage and removal of pus and toxin is still an important adjunct to treatment. Frequent stripping is commonly adivsed but perhaps not always carried out. Some veterinary practitioners still advocate surgical interference, providing no significant induration of the gland exists. This may be by complete amputation of the teat or by making a vertical incision down the teat barrel creating a fistula. Speed rather than surgical expertise is important.

Following infection during pregnancy, the subsequent offspring have been shown to have growth arrest lines and reduced thymus weights (Carole Richardson, 1982). Farmers have commented that calves born out of affected dams have not grown as well as their peers. The effect on the thymus may have an immunological implication.

Summer mastitis is usually defined as an infection of the non-lactating mammary gland during July, August and September. A condition with many clinical and bacteriological similarities occurred this year in a herd of milking cows in January in the north-west of England. All the bacteria associated with summer mastitis were identified in almost every case in various combinations. There were 184 cows in milk and 114 quarters were affected. The majority had only one quarter per cow, though multiple infections appeared more commonly later on. Five maiden heifers and one bull also developed infections.

Treatment with Metrinadazole and Penicillin by the intramammary route held the clinical signs, but relapses occurred immediately following the cessation of treatment. Subsequently, slaughter took place without treatment.

Two Mycoplasmas and one Acheloplasma have been associated with the disease outbreak. Despite extensive cultures of both milk and tissue, the isolation rate of these Mycoplasmas has remained extremely low. All the cows affected have remained serologically negative to Mycoplasmosis. The significance of these organisms remains unknown (Jasper, 1982). It was noted that at the time of the disease outbreak, nutritional, parasitological and milking machine problems were identified.

CHEMICAL FLY CONTROL ON CATTLE: RISKS FOR THE DEVELOPMENT OF RESISTANCE

R. De Deken

Instituut voor Tropische Geneeskunde,
"Prins Leopold",
Nationalestraat 155B, 2000 Antwerpen, Belgium.

ABSTRACT

Chemical fly control on heifers is frequently used in Europe as a preventive measure against summer mastitis. This paper warns against the potential development of resistance in cattle visiting flies, following the extensive use of insecticides. Several mechanisms of resistance have already been reported in *Haematobia irritans* from different parts of the U.S. Some recommendations are given in order to decrease the rate of development of resistance.

When dealing with the prevention of summer mastitis, a warning against the risks of developing resistance against chemical fly control is apparently not superfluous. Several species of flies such as *Lucilia cuprina, Chrysomia putoria, Cochliomyia hominivorax, Musca autumnalis* and *Haematobia irritans, i.e.* species visiting grazing ruminants, have been reported to develop resistance some time after remanent insecticides were used. (Busvine and Shanahan, 1961; Townsend and Busvine, 1969; Knap *et al.*, 1985; Nolan, 1985). These insecticides, whether in ear-tags or pour-on formulations are frequently used in Europe particularly for the prevention of summer mastitis in heifers.

The vectors of the summer mastitis pathogens, *i.e.* the *Hydroteae* species, are unlikely to develop rapid resistance against insecticides used for long term fly-control, because these flies visit cattle for a short time only, and even then, just stay on those parts of the body with a low concentration of insecticide, such as the udder region and around the eyes.

This is not so for *Haematobia irritans* however, a species frequently visiting cattle. In fact, resistance in *H. irritans* was first demonstrated in the south of the U.S.A. (McDuffie, 1960) where it is now known to occur after 2 to 4 years of intensive use of insecticidal ear-tags. The reasons for this are obvious:

— In these regions the climatic conditions are favourable for the reproduction of *Ha. irritans*, allowing development of several generations per year.

— A population of *Ha. irritans* is strictly confined to a particular herd with little or no immigration of susceptible individuals from another population. In such a population the selection pressure can be very high as ear-tags provide protection for 12 to 16 weeks and usually all animals are tagged.

— Furthermore, the blood sucking *Ha. irritans* remains on the animal for a long time, which facilitates picking up high doses of the insecticide. Therefore, all hornflies in the vicinity of a treated herd will come into contact with the insecticide and selection of resistant strains will proceed rapidly. For this reason we can expect that *Ha. irritans* will probably also be the first species of cattle visiting dipterians in Europe in which resistance develops. In the literature, resistance against the following insecticides has been reported in *Ha. irritans*:

Toxaphene (McDuffie, 1960); fenchlorphos (Burns and Wilson, 1963); fenvalerate (Schnitzerling *et al.*, 1982) with cross-resistance to DDT and cypermethrine; tetrachlorvinphos (Sheppard, 1983); fenvalerate (Sheppard, 1984) with cross-resistance to flucythrinate; permethrin and fenvalerate (Quisenberry *et al.*, 1984) with cross-resistance to cypermethrine, flucythrinate, DDT and deltamethrine (Byford *et al.*, 1985).

There are no observations of resistance against dichlorvos, probably because dichlorvos ear-tags are effective for 4 to 6 weeks only. The resistance against an insecticide does not need to be high at the time when the effect of the ear-tags has waned, *e.g.* the resistance in hornflies against tetrachlorvinphos had only a factor of 5 when the ear-tags became ineffective.

So far, in *Musca autumnalis* another cattle visiting fly, resistance has been observed only against methoxychlor (Knapp *et al.*, 1985).

The mechanisms through which resistance develops can be divided into four groups:

1. Behavioural resistance: when the insect avoids contact with the insecticide.
2. Decreased penetration: a gradually decreasing concentration of insecticide is able to penetrate the cuticle of the insect.
3. Increased detoxication or decreased activation of the insecticide: various enzymes in the insect are potentially responsible for this phenomenon. These include oxydases with mixed-function, hydrolases or glutathione-S-transferases.
4. The presence of chemical or physiological structures in the insect making them less susceptible to the action of the insecticide *e.g.*
   a) Acetylcholinesterases which are less inhibited by the organophosphates or carbamates. Such acetylcholinesterases give the metabolic enzymes more time to break down the insecticides.
   b) The "knock-down resistance", making the nerve fibres of the insect less susceptible to the action of pyrethroids and DDT.

So far, the mechanisms of resistance encountered in *Ha. irritans* are:

I. Behavioural resistance. In *Ha. irritans* this is based on:
   (i) Hypersensibility. A resistant population shows a higher level of irritability than a susceptible population to concentrations of an insecticide irritant to both populations.
   (ii) Lowered sensitivity threshold. Resistant individuals are irritated by concentrations of insecticides, which do not effect susceptible flies.

The occurrence of these mechanisms are illustrated by an observation of Lockwood *et al.* (1985). A population of *Ha. irritans* showed knock-down resistance against permethrin, fenvalerate, deltamethrin, cypermethrin and DDT, and had behavioural resistance to fenvalerate and permethrin, both the only two insecticides with which this strain had actually been in contact. The form of behavioural resistance to permethrin was different from that to fenvalerate. In the case of permethrin it was due to a lowered sensitivity threshold, in the case of fenvalerate it was due to hypersensitivity.

II. Metabolic resistance: Resistance in a strain of *Ha. irritans* (Red River) was partially abolished by piperonylbutoxide and DEF, two synergists. This suggests that some oxydases and esterases are partially responsible for the insusceptibility in this strain to pyrethroids. (Byford *et al.*, 1985).

III. Knock-down resistance was found in strains of *Ha. irritans*, with a broad cross-resistance to several pyrethroids and DDT. (Byford *et al.*, 1985). These examples illustrate that resistance against fly controlling chemicals might cause problems.

In order to decrease the rate of development of resistance, the following recommendations might be considered.

— The removal of all ear-tags at the end of the fly season when release of insecticide is decreasing and may allow the flies to survive subtoxic levels of insecticide.

— Insecticidal pour-on formulations should be renewed regularly, insuring an optimal level of insecticide on the animal.

It is important that the development of other methods for fly-control should be stimulated. In particular, the use of traps with odour baits, attractive to flies might be a rewarding topic for further research.

REFERENCES

Aehnelt, E. 1955. Zur Vorbeuge der Pyogenes-Mastitis bei Weiderindern mit Kontaktinsektiziden. Dtsch. tierärztl. Wochenschr., 62, 493-498.

Annual report Danish Pest Infestation Laboratory, 1985, DK 2800, Lyngby, Denmark.

Bahr, L. 1955. Continuous investigations concerning summer mastitis in dry cows. Anden meddelelse. Dansk Månedsskr. Dyrl., 63, 365-388.

Bech-Nielsen, S., Bornstein, S., Christensson, D., Wallgren, T., and Zakrisson, G. 1982. *Parafilaria bovicola* (Tubangui, 1934) in cattle: Epizootiology – Vector studies and experimental transmission of *Parafilaria bovicola* to cattle. Am. J. Vet. Res., 43 (6), 948-954.

Beimgraben, J. 1983. Untersuchungen zur Prophylaxe der enzootischen Pyogenes Mastitis in Praxisbetrieben Schleswig-Holstein. Vet. med. Diss. Hannover.

Bertels, G., and Robijns, J.M. 1983. Prevention of summer mastitis in cattle by fly control: A field trial with permethrin and cypermethrin. Vlaams Diergeneesk. Tijdschr., 52 (2), 77-87.

Bramley, A.J., Hillerton, J.E., Higgs, T.M. and Hogben, E.M. 1985. The carriage of summer mastitis pathogens by muscoid flies. British Vet. J., 141, 618.

Brown, J.F., and Adkins, T.R., 1972. Relationship of feeding activity of face fly (*Musca autumnalis* DeGeer) to production of keratoconjunctivitis in calves. Am. J. Vet. Res., 33, 2551-2555.

Burns, E.C. and Wilson, B.H. 1963. Field resistance of horn flies to the organic phosphate insecticide Ronnel. J. Econ. Entomol., 56, 718.

Büscher, D. 1975. Praxiserfahrung bei ter Therapie der sogenannten holsteinischen Euterseuche (Pyogenes Mastitis des Rindes) unter besonderer Berücksichtigung der Anwendung von Ubrocelan. Prakt.Tierarzt, 6, 348-350.

Busvine, J.R. and Shanahan, G.J. 1961. The resistance spectrum of a dieldrin-resistant strain of the blowfly *(Lucilia cuprina)*. Entomol. Exp. Appl., 4, 1.

Byford, R.L., Quisenberry, S.S., Sparks, T.C. and Lockwood, J.A. 1985. Spectrum of insecticide cross-resistance in pyrethroid-resistant populations of *Haematobia irritans* (Diptera: Muscidae). J. Econ. Entomol., 78, 768.

Cornelisse, J.L., Saes, J.M.F. and Atteveld, J.C. 1970. De isolatie van anaerobe streptococcen, peptostreptococcen, uit uiersecretum van runderen met wrang, Tijdschr. Diergeneesk., 95, 387-391.

Dieckerhoff, W. 1878. Die zu Stendorff in Holstein herrschende infectiöse Euterentzündung der Kühe. Wochenschr. Tierheilk. Viehzucht, 21, 97-102.

Dommerholt, G.J.G. Acute zomermastitis (zomerwrang): een gecompliceerd probleem. referaat C.H.K.S. Dronten, Gezondheidsdienst voor Dieren in Overijssel te Zwolle, Oktober 1985.

Edmonds, M.J. and Welsch, J.A. 1979. The prevention of summer mastitis in dry cows by intramammary infusions of ampicillin and cloxacillen, Vet. Rec., 104, 554-555.

Elger, D. 1985. Untersuchungen zur Biologie und Ökologie symboviner Musciden un Tabaniden in Norddeutschland (Diptera: Muscidae, Tabanidae) Thesis, Univ. Hannover.

Elger, D. and Liebisch, A. 1982. Felduntersuchungen zur Wirksamkeit von Permethrin zur Bekämpfung von Fliegen an Weiderindern in Norddeutschland. Tierärztl. Umschau, 37, 437-442.

Gezondheidsdienst voor Dieren in Overijssel. 1986. 38e Jaarverslag, 29-31.

Götze, R. 1951. Zur Bekämpfung der Euterentzündung des Rindes. Dtsch. tierärztl. Wochenschr., 58, 198-205.

Hammer, O. 1941. Biological and ecological investigations on flies associated with pasturing cattle and their excrement. Vidensk. Meddr. Dansk Naturh. Fore., **105**, 141-393.

Hillerton, J.E., Bramley, A.J. and Broom, D.M. 1983. *Hydrotaea irritans* and summer mastitis in calves. Vet. Rec., **113**, 88.

Hillerton, J.E., Bramley, A.J. and Yarrow, N.H. 1985. Control of flies (Diptera: Muscidae) on dairy heifers by Flectron® ear-tags. Brit. Vet. J., **141** (2), 160-167.

Hillerton, J.E., Bramley, A.J. and Yarrow, N.H. Control of flies (Diptera: Muscidae) on dairy heifers by Flectron® ear tags. Brit. Vet. J. – in press.

Hillerton, J.E., Broom, D.M., Bramley, A.J. and Watson, C.A. 1982. *Hydrotaea irritans* ♀'s in the transmission of summer mastitis. Proceedings R.A.M.C. Millbank. Ectoparasites of Veterinary and Medical importance in temperate areas.

Heidrich, H.J., Fiebiger, E. 1964. Untersuchungen über die Pyogenes Mastitis des Rindes mit besonderer Berücksichtigung der Fermenttherapie: I. Berl. und Münch. Tierärztl. Wschr. **77**, 234-236.

Heidrich, H.J. Fiebiger, E. 1965. Untersuchungen über die Pyogenes Mastitis des Rindes mit besonderer Berücksichtigung der Fermenttherapie: II. Berl. und Münch. Tierärztl. Wschr. **78**, 341-342.

Hofmann, W. 1985. Erfahrungen mit dem Einsatz von insekticidhaltigen Ohrmarken zur Fliegenabwehr bei Weiderindern. Dtsch. tierärztl. Wochenschr., **92**, 353-356.

Jasper, D.E. 1982. The role of Mycoplasma in bovine mastitis. J. A. V. M. A., **181**, 158-162.

Jespersen, J.B. 1981. Ecological studies on the insect fauna on pasturing heifers, with special reference to the transmission of summer mastitis. Report, University of Aarhus, Department of Zoology, 70 pp.

Jespersen, J.B. 1984. Flies on grazing cattle. Danish Pest Inf. Lab. Ann. Rep. 1983 (1984), 51-54.

Jespersen, J.B. and Vagn-Jensen, K.-M. 1985. Flies on grazing cattle: Field evaluation of ear-tags and collars for fly and disease control. Danish Pest Inf. Lab. Ann. Rep. 1984 (1985), 52-62.

Jespersen, J.B. and Vagn-Jensen, K.-M. 1986. Flies on grazing cattle and horses. Danish Pest Inf. Lab. Ann. Rep. 1985 (1986), 59-67.

Jespersen, J.B., Nielsen, S. Achim, Vagn-Jensen, K.-M. and Nielsen, B. Overgaard. 1986. The spatial distribution of species of Diptera over the bodies of pasturing heifers in Denmark (in prep.).

Klastrup, N.O. 1983. Prophylactic methods available and recommended today. Proc. Heifer Mastitis Seminar, Stockholm-Helsinki.

Knapp, F.W., Herald, F. and Schwinghammer, K.A. 1985. Comparative toxicity of selected insecticides to laboratory-reared and field-collected face flies. J. Econ. Entomol., **78**, 860-862.

Künast, C., Schäfer, B., Schmelz, H. and Schah-Zeidi, M. 1983. Untersuchungen über die Kontrolle von Dipteren an Weide vieh in Süddeutschland durch cypermethrinhaltige Ohrmarken. Berl. Münch. Tierärztl. Wochenschr., **96**, 131-134.

Liebisch, A. 1983 a. Parasitenbekämpfung in der Rinderpraxis, Teil 1: Fliegenbekämpfung bei Weiderindern. Milchpraxis, **21**, 44-46.

Liebisch, A. 1983 b. Parasitenbekämpfung in der Rinderpraxis, Teil 2: Neue Methoden der Fliegenbekämpfung zur Verbeuge der Sommer-mastitis bei Färsen. Milchpraxis, **21**, 120-122.

Liebisch, A. 1984. Fliegen und Bremsen bei Weiderindern. deren Bedeutung und die Möglichkeiten zur Bekämpfung. Milchpraxis, **22**, 140-142.

Liebisch, A. 1985. Untersuchungen über die langzeitwirkung insektizidhaltiger Ohrmarken (Permethrin und Cypermethrin) zur Bekämpfung von Fliegen und Bremsen bei Weiderindern in Norddeutschland. Dtsch. tierärztl. Wochenschr., **92**, 186-191.

Liebisch, A. 1986. Weidefliegen jetzt strategisch bekämpfen. Top Agrar, 6. Juni 1986 (Rind), 14-16.

Liebisch, A. and Elger, D. 1983. Weidefliegen und deren Bekämpfung bei Rindern. Fortschritte der Veterinärmedizin, Heft 37: 15. Kongressbericht. 267.

Lindloff, G. 1958. Euterbesprühung mit den Kontaktinsektiziden DDT und Toxaphen-Lindan zur Mastitisprophylaxe der Weiderinder. Teil 2 Thesis, Hannover, Tierärztliche Hochschule.

Lockwood, J.A., Byford, R.L., Story, R.N., Sparks, T.C. and Quisenberry, S.S. 1985. Behavioural resistance to the pyrethroids in the horn fly, *Haematobia irritans* (Diptera: Muscidae). Environ. Entomol., **14**, 873-880.

Malze, A. 1957. Euterbesprühungen mit den Kontaktinsektiziden DDT und Toxaphen-Lindan zur Mastitis-Prophylaxe der Weiderinder. Teil 1 Thesis, Hannover, Tierärztliche Hochschule.

McDuffie, W.C., 1960. Current status of insecticide resistance in livestock pests. Misc. Publ. Entomol. Soc. Am., **2**, 49-54.

Nielsen, —. 1908. Eine neue Euterseuche in Schleswig-Holstein. Berl. tierärztl. Wochenschr. **24**, 969-970.

Nielsen, B. Overgaard, 1971. Some observations on biting Midges (Diptera: Ceratopogonidae) attacking grazing cattle in Denmark. Ent. Scand., **2**, 94-98.

Nielsen, B. Overgaard, Nielsen, B.M. and Christensen, O. 1971. Contributions to the biology of the plantation fly, *Hydrotaea irritans* Fall. Ent. Meddr., **39**, 30-44.

Nielsen, B. Overgaard, Nielsen, B.M. and Christensen, O. 1972. The plantation fly, *Hydrotaea irritans* Fall., on grazing heifers. Ent. Meddr., **40**, 151-173.

Nielsen, B. Overgaard and Christensen, O. 1975. A mass attack by the biting Midge *Culicoides nubeculosus* (Mg.) (Diptera: Ceratopogonidae) on grazing cattle in Denmark. A new aspect of sewage discharge. Nord. Vet. Med., **27**, 365-372.

Nielsen, B. Overgaard, Jespersen, J.B. and Nielsen, S. Achim. 1986. The fauna of Diptera attacking pasturing heifers in Denmark (in prep.).

Nolan, J. 1985. Mechanisms of resistance to chemicals in arthropod parasites of veterinary importance. Vet. Parasit., **18**, 155-166.

O'Rourke, D.J.O., Chamings, R.J. and Booth, J.M. 1985. Summer mastitis incidence: 1978-83. Vet. Rec., **115**, 62-63.

Pearson, J.K.L. 1951. Further experiments in the use of penicillin in the prevention of *C. pyogenes*-infection of the non-lactating bovine udder. Vet. Rec., **68**, 215-220.

Pecheur, M. 1985. Protection of cattle against flies: use of cypermethrin impregnated ear-tags. Ann. Med. Vet., **129** (3), 215-218.

Petersen, A. 1924. Contributions to the natural history of the Danish Simuliidae. Kgl. danske Vidensk. Selsk. Skr., Naturvidensk. og Matematisk afd., 8. raekke **4**, 235-340.

Quisenberry, S.S., Lockwood, J.A., Byford, R.L., Wilson, H.K. and Sparks, T.C. 1984. Pyrethroid resistance in the horn fly, *Haematobia irritans*. J. Econ. Entomol., **77**, 1095-1098.

Reimers, H. 1888. Eutererkrankungen bei Weidekühen. Berl. tierärztl. Wochenschr., **4**, 18-20.

Richardson, Carole. 1982. Proc. Biuatrics Conf. Amsterdam.

Saes, J.M.F. 1971. Occurrence, pathogenesis and control of bovine *C. pyogenes*-mastitis (summer mastitis) in the province of Limburg. Tijdschr. Diergeneesk., **96**, 1306-1317.

Schmidt, C.D., Kunz, S.E., Petersen, H.D. and Robertson, J.L. 1985. Resistance of horn flies (Diptera: Muscidae) to permethrin and fenvalerate. J. Econ. Entomol., **78** (2), 402-406.

Schnitzerling, H.J., Noble, P.J., MacQueen, A. and Dunham, R.J. 1982. Resistance of the buffalo fly, *Haematobia irritans exigua* (De Meyere), to two synthetic pyrethroids and DDT. J. Austr. Entomol. Soc., **21**, 77-80.

Sheppard, D.C. 1983. Stirofos resistance in a population of horn flies. J. Georgia Entomol. Soc., **18**, 370-376.

Sheppard, D.C. 1984. Fenvalerate and flucythrinate resistance in a horn fly, *Haematobia irritans*, population selected with fenvalerate. J. Agric. Entomol., **1**, 305-310.

Sol, J. and Vardy, A. 1982. Effect of and length of protection offered by Cepravin Dry Cow in the prevention of summer mastitis. Tijdschr. Diergeneesk., **107**, 466-474.

Sol, J. 1983. Summer Mastitis: Pathogenesis, losses, incidence and prevention. Tijdschr. Diergeneesk., **108**, 443-452.

Sol, J. 1984. Control methods in summer mastitis: the importance of fly control. Proc. XIIIth World Congress on Diseases of Cattle, 236-242, Durban, S.A.

Sol, J., Vecht, U. and Thomas, G. 1985. Summer mastitis: incidence, bacteriology, etiology, methods of prevention and entomological aspects. Kiel. Milch. Forschung., **37**, 593-600.

Sorensen, G. Hoi. 1974. Studies on the aetiology and transmission of summer mastitis. Nord. Vet. Med., **26**, 122-132.

Sparks, T.C., Quisenberry, S.S., Lockwood, J.A., Byford, R.L. and Roush, R.T. 1985. Insecticide resistance in the horn fly, *Haematobia irritans*. J. of Agric. Entomol., **2** (3), 217-233.

Tarry, D.W., Wilson, C.D. and Stuart, P. 1978. The headfly *Hydrotaea irritans* and summer mastitis infection. Vet. Rec., **102**, 91.

Taylor, S.M., Mallon, T. and Blanchflower, J. 1935. Effect of flycythrinate impregnated ear-tags on fly attack in cattle. Vet. Rec., **116**, 566-567.

Thomsen, M. 1938. The housefly *(Musca domestica)* and the stable fly *(Stomoxys calcitrans)*. 176de beretning fra forsogslaboratoriet. 352 pp. Copenhagen.

Titchener, R.N. and Cochrane, D.G. 1980. Use of pyrethroids. Vet. Rec., **106**, 517.

Tolle, A., Reichmuth, J., Franke, V. and Beimgraben, J. 1985. Untersuchungen zur Pyogenes-Mastitis des Rindes, Kieler Milchwirtschaftliche Forschungsberichte, **36**, 125-212.

Townsend, M.G. and Busvine, J.R. 1969. The mechanism of malathion resistance in the blowfly, *Chrysomia putoria*. Entomol. Exp. Appl., **12**, 243-267.

Ussing, Hj. 1925. Faunistic and biological contributions to the natural history of the Danish Simuliidae. Vidensk. Medd. fra Dansk Naturh. Foren., **80**, 517-542.

Weigt, U. and Lindfeld, A. 1976. Möglichkeiten zur Verhütung der Sommermastitis. Milch-praxis, **14**, 10-12.

Weitz, B. 1949. *C. pyogenes* infection in cattle with special reference to summer mastitis. Vet. Rec., **61**, 123-126.

Wright, C.L., Titchener, R.N. and Hughes, J. 1984. Insecticidal ear-tags and sprays for the control of flies on cattle. Vet. Rec., **115** (3), 60-62.

Yeoman, G.H. and Warren, B.C. 1984. Summer mastitis. Br. Vet. J., **140**, 232-243.

DISCUSSION

The discussion opened with a short exchange of comments regarding the success of therapeutic treatment of summer mastitis cases. Although some successful therapy results were reported in the introductory talk to the session, where complete functional recovery of the udder tissue was obtained in a high percentage of cases, the general experience of the participants working in this field was that the quarter is usually lost to milk production. The possibility was then raised that poor recovery might be due to the timing of therapy after onset of infection and the question phrased as to how soon after illness appears should treatment be applied. Unfortunately, there appeared to be a lack of information regarding this point. Field observations suggest that the udder is hard and swollen after 12 hrs but care should be taken before accepting this as the norm as authentication is difficult. The results of infection experiments carried out in The Netherlands showed that clear clinical signs are present 4 hours after injecting pathogens. Even here however, care should be taken before drawing any conclusions as early signs are not a key to prognosis. The general advice given was that treatment should be carried out as soon as any indication of summer mastitis is seen.

The remainder of the discussion centred on summer mastitis prevention. Firstly, the suggestion was made that more attention should be given to immuno-prophylaxis. After this efficacy, mode of working and potential drawbacks of fly control were considered.

As far as efficacy is concerned early application of ear-tags was concluded to be preferable to later application. This was true for all flies, including *Hydrotaea irritans* but particularly for *Haematobia irritans*. The question was then raised as to whether ear-tags and pour-ons achieved control of *H. irritans* directly or indirectly as a result of controlling biting flies such as *Haem. irritans*. Although the numbers of both species are reduced by fly control it is difficult to uncouple the direct/indirect hypothesis. One of the reasons underlying this is the paucity of information regarding the behaviour and interactions between the two species. Experiments carried out in the U.K. where ear-tags were removed from cattle where excellent fly control had been achieved resulted in rapid return and sustained high fly challenge of *H. irritans* and *Morellia simplex* but no return of biting flies whatsoever. It was suggested that this could have resulted from a behavioural resistance or reduced effect on these sucking flies, which are not obligatory symbovine flies. Similar effects were also reported from Belgium with experiments carried out using pour-on formulations. The direct/indirect mechanism of action still remains to be resolved although the experience of the Danish researchers was that if one could not control the biting fly species then no success was achieved in controlling *Hydrotaea irritans*.

This latter point raises one potential future problem. When, as in other countries, resistance develops in the horn fly population then this will result in no control of *H. irritans*.

It is thus essential to resolve the indirect/direct hypothesis mentioned above.

Finally, information was requested regarding the residue and persistance characteristics of the insecticides used for fly control not only with regard to deposition in the animal but also with regard to environmental pollution. As far as the technique used for application is concerned the advice given was that the amount of insecticide deposited in the environment was generally less with ear-tags than with pour-ons. However, pyrethroids from ear-tags can cause a problem when these are lost, as the amount of insecticide remaining even at the end of the season can be considerable — up to 50% of the original amount. In addition to some of the pour-on ending up in the soil during application there is also a considerable potential risk from disposal of what is left over after treatment has been carried out, in many cases this is simply poured away. The newly developed feed through application can result in environmental problems as the insecticide is excreted in the faeces. As far as residues are concerned, information was presented indicating that deltamethrin can be absorbed and care must be taken to avoid toxicological problems. Pyrethroids can be recovered in small quantities in milk: tests indicate that diazinon and organophosphate are also recoverable from milk but generally in such small amounts as to be acceptable. However, this is not the case in the latter when that milk is used to make cheese products and the amount of fat in the product is higher than 10%.

6. ECONOMICS AND ERGONOMICS

Chairmen J. Reichmuth & G. Bertels

ECONOMIC AND ERGONOMIC IMPLICATIONS OF SUMMER MASTITIS

J. Reichmuth

Institut für Hygiene,
Bundesanstalt für Milchforschung,
D 2300 Kiel, F.R.G.

ABSTRACT

Every case of summer mastitis causes an economic loss which can be evaluated individually and ranges between 250,-- and 3000,-- DM depending on the value of the animal and the seriousness of the disease. In Schleswig-Holstein, Federal Republic of Germany, the average loss per case is assumed to be approximately 1000,-- DM. There exists a variety of preventive measures, such as antibiotic treatments, insecticide treatments differing in formulation and duration of effectiveness (one to four applications per animal and season may be necessary), protection of the teat orifice with adhesive plaster, keeping the animals at risk indoors or sending them to areas known for a low incidence of summer mastitis. Costs of material and expenditure of work tend to be somewhat inversely proportional and are prone to local variations. A simple formula is given to approximate the marginal costs of prevention reasonable for a predicted incidence on the individual farm. The crucial point is the limited information of the incidence in the past as a parameter for the risk in the season to come, for there are considerable differences in incidence between years. It rests with the farmer according to his mentality to choose preventive measures which use the whole expenditure at the beginning of the season (*e.g.* ear-tags, antibiotic treatment) or to prefer a method which allows for preventive treatment only when the risk of the disease is expected to grow due to weather conditions (*e.g.* pour-on insecticides). In the latter decision he has to face the risk of being late and other urgent work (*e.g.* harvesting) might interfere.

INTRODUCTION

If summer mastitis occurs, the economic loss is considerable. On the other hand the measures available to prevent this disease to a reasonable extent need relatively high expenditure of material and/or work per animal and season.

This paper deals with some economic and ergonomic deliberations how to decide on the appropriate approach for the individual farm.

ECONOMIC VALUATION OF THE DISEASE

Every case of summer mastitis causes an economic damage which can be evaluated individually and ranges between 250,-- and 3000,-- DM or even more, depending on the value of the animal and the seriousness of the disease. This comprises partial or total loss of the animal, costs of attempts at therapy and negative effects on breeding process. In Schleswig-Holstein, Federal Republic of Germany, the average loss per case is assumed to be approximately 1000,-- DM.

Since 1978, all cases of summer mastitis in yield controlled herds are registered. The

196

results are shown in Figure 1 (Tolle and Reichmuth, 1985).

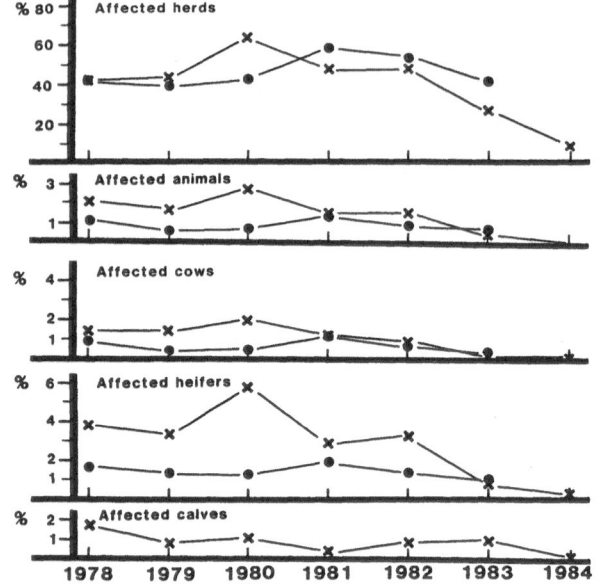

Fig. 1. Incidence of Summer mastitis
Schleswig-Holstein, FRG: x——x
England and Wales (MMB): ●——●

The number of cases ranged between 15,000 (2.7%) in 1980 and 900 (0.2%) in 1984. Yield control organization covers approximately 50% of all dairy herds in Schleswig-Holstein. Taking into account these figures the total economic damage in this part of Germany can be estimated between 30 and 1.8 million DM respectively.

The broad variation in the economic importance of this disease within only four years was of influence on official as well as on private interest in summer mastitis.

In 1986 the situation was still near that of 1984, and thus summer mastitis does not now play an important role among the actual problems in dairying.

PREVENTIVE MEASURES — EXPENDITURE AND ERGONOMICS

There exists a variety of preventive measures such as antibiotic treatments, insecticide treatments differing in formulation and duration of effectiveness, protection of the teat orifice with adhesive plaster, keeping the animals at risk indoors or sending them to areas known for a low incidence of summer mastitis.

The expenditure for preventive measures in a season consists of the price for the drugs, the amortization of installations and devices for application *e.g.* corrals for rounding up, summer mastitis drinking box, spray pump etc. and costs for labour and transport.

Costs of material and expenditure of work tend to be somewhat inversely proportional and are prone to local variations.

Under practical farming conditions a pure economic decision towards the lowest total expenditure for the treatment per animal is not always feasible: the timing of treatment must fit into the sequence of other operations on the farm. Thus the ergonomic preference may overrule the economic one.

Under these considerations it can be expected, that any measure is preferred which can be carried out before pasturing in spring, because of the easier handling of the animals in the stable and a sufficient manpower at the time. This procedure implies, however, that the whole expenditure for prevention is invested at one time, when actual risk for summer mastitis in the season to come is only a guess. It rests with the mentality of the farmer, to choose this alternative or to prefer a method which allows for preventive treatment only when the risk of the disease is expected to increase due to weather conditions. In this case he has to face the danger of being too late and other urgent work (e.g. harvesting) might interfere.

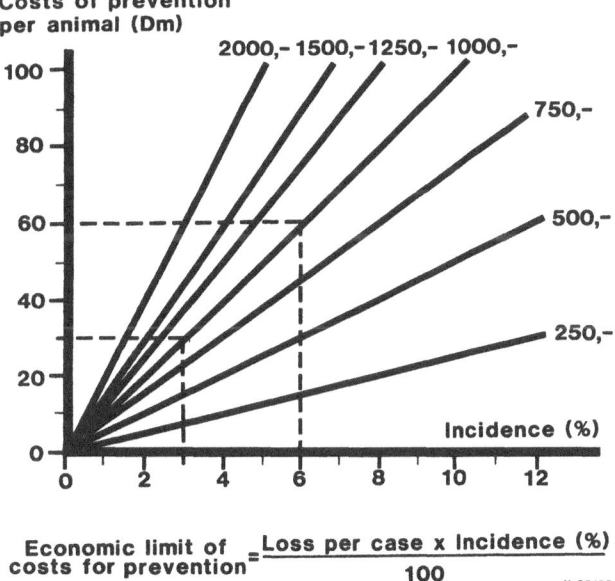

Fig. 2. Model for the evaluation of economic limits for the prevention of summer mastitis.

CONCLUSION

Besides the ergonomic considerations the incidence of summer mastitis in an area or a farm in the last year(s) is the basis for the decision on the reasonable level of expenditure for prevention for the season to come.

In Figure 2 a formula is given which leads to the marginal costs of prevention per animal and year in relation to the estimated incidence and the average economic loss per case.

The graph is the transformation of the formula into several levels of damage.

Example: let the incidence be 3% and the loss per case DM 1000,--, then an expenditure for prevention up to DM 30 per animal may be reasonable.

Regarding the tendency of incidence in the last years (Fig. 1) it has to be kept in mind, that this approach under the actual situation leads to a rather low threshold for seasonable costs of prevention per animal, which is below the cheapest measure.

CONSEQUENCES OF SUMMER MASTITIS ON DAIRY FARM PRODUCTIVITY

J.W. Seinhorst

Proefstation v.d. Rundveehouderij,
Runderweg 6, 8219 PK Lelystad, The Netherlands

ABSTRACT

Farming in an area where summer mastitis is endemic means a higher risk of loosing young stock.

The number of animals that will be affected by summer mastitis during one season can not be predicted, not even approximately. So the farmer tends to take measures every year to minimize losses at a level that reasonable losses can be overcome. Farming for optimal results depends on a number of factors such as: area, land situation, number of cows, amount of labour, milk-quotum, milk price, etc.

Adapting farming to the risk of summer mastitis means that from an economical point of view the optimal farming situation is not achieved. Compared to summer mastitis-free areas this means a lower income. This is so for years without summer mastitis. In years where animals are affected by summer mastitis, extra financial losses, such as reduced value of affected animals, are added to the already existing losses.

As costs, related to farming in summer mastitis-areas, are different for every farm situation, it is not possible to give an overall figure. More detailed calculations have to be made. On the other hand a farmer is willing to spend some money on prevention of summer mastitis to relieve his mind from a constant burden.

The number of animals affected by summer mastitis varies from year to year in the Netherlands. Hence, the financial losses, based on estimates, range from 6 to 60 million dutch guilders per year. Only the reduced value of affected animals and costs for treatment are incorporated in this figure.

However, farming in an area where summer mastitis is endemic means a higher risk of losing animals. The number of animals that will be affected by summer mastitis during one season cannot be predicted, not even approximately. The farmer therefore tends to take measures every year to minimize the risk at such a level that losses can be compensated within reasonable limits. The strategy chosen by the farmer will largely depend on the existence of other possibilities of raising young stock, without putting them at risk to summer mastitis. Adaptation of farming to the risk of summer mastitis means that in a large number of situations an optimal farming situation may not be achieved from an economical point of view.

The number of possibilities from which a farmer can choose is limited. The main situations are:

1. grazing of young stock in summer mastitis areas
2. grazing of young stock in summer mastitis free areas
3. housing of young stock during the summer period.

Farming for optimal results depends on a number of factors, related to farming conditions. Such factors are: area, land-situation, number of dairy cows, stocking rate, amount of labour available, mechanisation, investment, milk price and milk-quotum etc.

Situations 2 and 3 can be a combination of farm situation and measures against summer mastitis.

For instance: a farm with a high stocking rate can graze its young stock elsewhere. Extra costs are incured by transport of cattle.

or: in a situation where grazing of young stock near the farm is difficult, the farmer can chose for zero-grazing.

If grazing young stock in an endemic summer mastitis area is the only possibility for the farmer, the economical consequences can be rather large. In such a situation the farmer raises more young stock. In fact, the farmer is forced to choose the level of young stock about 12 — 15 months before the problems can occur. Depending on what will happen, the farmer is faced with a number of situations.

Schematically this can be approached as follows:

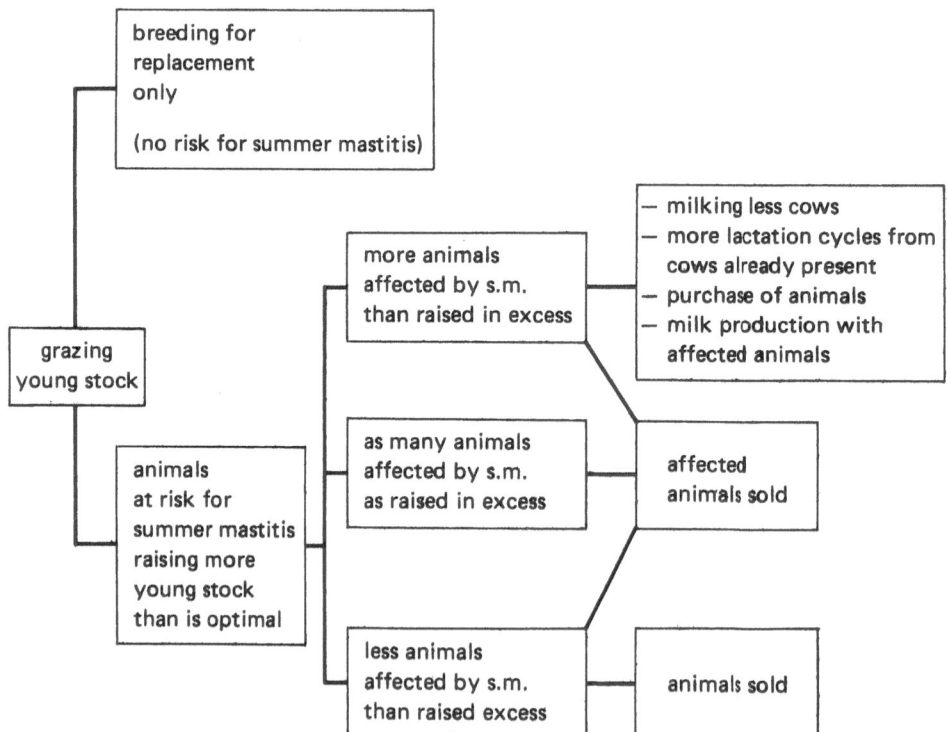

In addition to this in all situations where summer mastitis occurs, additional costs will arise such as:

— costs for treatment incured from visits by the veterinairian, antibiotics, labour,

— reduced value of affected animals,

— possible loss of breeding value because daughters of sires with a high breeding value can be affected to a higher extent.

A good prognosis and recovery for affected animals (certainly in the case of other kinds of mastitis) can reduce a certain amount of the costs initially calculated.

The costs that are a consequence of raising more young stock than is needed for replacement lowers the income of the farmer (see Fig. 1). The level of income depends on the farm situation.

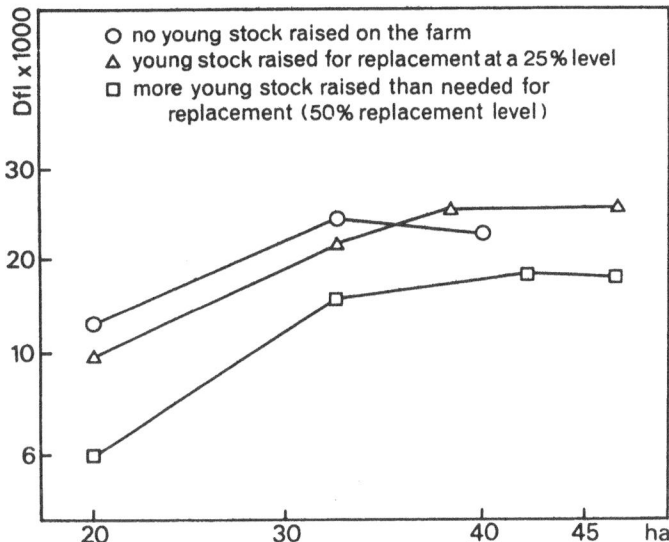

Fig. 1. Relation between income in Dfl x 1000 and area in hectares at different levels of raising young stock (source M.L. Douna, 1972).
Note: Allthough the income- and cost figures of the calculations leading to this graph are not up to date, the trends in this graph are still valid. More up to date information (influence of milk quotum incorporated) was not available. The graph presented refers to a one man farm situation ("family" farm).

When a farmer decides to raise more young stock there are three contingencies that must be considered if summer mastitis cases occur:

a) more animals are affected than are raised in excess

consequences: — milk production is lower because there are less animals to replace culled cows,

— milk production has to be maintained with older cows that otherwise would have been culled,

— animals have to be purchased. The price to be paid can increase because of a lack of animals.

all consequences increase costs.

b) as many animals are affected as are raised in excess

    consequences: — "none".

c) less animals are affected than are raised in excess

    consequences: — animals have to be sold. The price can be lower because there is a surplus of animals on the market.

To produce reliable and up to date figures on costs of summer mastitis, calculations have to be made. The best method for such a problem is the so called "linear programming" approach. On the other hand, it can be stated that costs for raising extra young stock are so high that the alternative, a reliable prevention method, can certainly be more economical. And last of all, the farmer is no longer worried by the fact that he does not know the number of animals he might lose during the next summer season.

ECONOMIC LOSSES ASSOCIATED WITH SUMMER MASTITIS
IN PREGNANT AND NON—PREGNANT HEIFERS

P. Nansen*, J.W. Hansen**, V. Oestergaard***

*Royal Veterinary and Agricultural University,
13 Bülowsvej, DK—1870 Frederiksberg C., Denmark.
**College of Veterinary Medicine,
Virginia Tech, Blacksburg, Virginia 24061, U.S.A.
***National Institute of Animal Science,
Foulum, DK—8830 Oerum Soenderlyng, Denmark.

ABSTRACT

In Denmark, the economical losses associated with summer mastitis are mainly due to an irreversible destruction of lactating glands of heifers. In the present investigation we followed the fate of pregnant and non-pregnant Black-Pied Friesian heifers after their initial acute disease contracted while grazing on common grasslands in northern Jutland. For the pregnant heifer the average loss was 5,800 Dkr. (1984). This was primarily explained by a reduction in the expected milk yield due to early slaughtering resulting in a shortened lactation period due to failure of the affected gland to produce milk. For the non-pregnant heifer the average loss of 2,000 Dkr. (1984) was also mainly attributable to slaughtering at an early stage, *i.e.* 4 months (average) after the attack. In both categories of heifers, deaths, treatment costs, transport costs, *etc.* played a relatively insignificant part in the overall losses. The ongoing genetically-governed increase of performance was believed to be diminished by the unintended early removal of recruitment stock. Attempts were made to estimate losses at the herd level. Cost/benefit outcomes resulting from various preventive strategies were dependent on levels of incidence in the herd.

INTRODUCTION

Attempts to estimate the economical losses brought about by summer mastitis in cattle have been made in a number of investigations in Denmark and other European countries. In most studies, estimations have mainly been based on information about the direct consequences of the clinical outbreak(s), and the overall losses have been calculated out of this. Only few investigations have followed and analyzed the fate of the affected animal after its general health restoration. However, this is essential because — though the animal may be in a good condition — the invalidated and non-productive gland calls for decision making depending on herd management practices *etc.*

In a comprehensive epidemiological study involving cattle on permanent grazing in northern Jutland (Denmark) we demonstrated that animals of the Black-Pied Friesian breed were clearly more predisposed than other breeds, and that pregnant heifers, in particular those towards the end of the gestation period, were at a significantly higher risk than non-pregnant heifers (Kronborg *et al.*, 1985; Madsen *et al.*, 1986).

In the present investigation we followed in some detail affected Black-Pied Friesian heifers from the onset of acute disease until their death or dismissal from the herd. The study, which was initiated in 1981 in and around Store Vildmose, northern Jutland, included pregnant as well as non-pregnant heifers. All animals involved in the study showed the manifest disease picture described and classified by Hoi Sorensen (1979) as summer mastitis.

MATERIALS AND METHODS

Pre-classified questionnaires were used. Information was sought through an initial questionnaire in July-August-September 1981 in association with the clinical outbreaks — and subsequently through questionnaires sent to the farmers at intervals up to April 1983. The investigation comprised full description on 113 heifers, of which 79 were pregnant and 34 were non-pregnant. Only a few animals could not be followed, because of incomplete information or lack of farmers collaboration. Data obtained by the questionnaires together with information directly obtainable from the disease registrations at Store Vildmose and from associated veterinary practitioners provided us with information about: age of animals at the time of the disease outbreak, stage of pregnancy at the time of the outbreak, course of disease, medical and surgical treatment, extra labour required in association with handling of diseased animals, transport of animal to farm and stable-feeding during the grazing season, data on dismissed animals (time of death, slaughtering, carcass quality *etc.*), calving time. In addition, approximate estimates were made on the following: animal weights, milk yields and weight gains up to slaughtering, feed consumptions, labour investments in the stable, *etc.*

The economical loss per animal was estimated by comparing average costs and yields of affected animals with those of non-affected animals. The latter data were from Black-Pied Friesian cattle, obtained by i.a. Oestergaard (1983 a, b).

RESULTS AND DISCUSSION

Pregnant heifers

The average age of the 79 animals at the time of the acute disease was 716 days and the calculated average weight 400 kg. Veterinary medical expenses, costs of extra labour, transport and stable-feeding during the grazing season made up a total of 336 Dkr. (1984) per animal. Table 1 shows the most essential economical results from animals with and without summer mastitis followed to the end of the first lactation period at which time all affected heifers had been done away with.

Out of the affected animals 1% died, 23% were slaughtered before calving while the remaining 76% were sent to slaughter from the time of calving and successively onwards. The average length of their lactation period was 125 days (as opposed to 210 days for the 19% of heifers without summer mastitis that for some reason or other also leave the milking herd after their first lactation). When yields of affected and non-affected animals are compared the most conspicuous difference is the average income from milk production. This may be explained by differences in the number of pregnant animals entering lactation, length of lactation periods and daily yields. It has been demonstrated that failure of one quarter to produce milk usually lowers the total milk yield by approximately 15%.

TABLE 1. Calculation of loss per pregnant heifer (followed to the end of first lactation)

	Summer mastitis infected		Non-infected	
Incomes				
Dead	0.01 x 400 kg x 0.60 Dkr :	2	0.01 x 400 kg x 0.60 Dkr :	2
Slaughtered before calving	0.23 x 450 kg x 12.00 Dkr :	1,242	0.03 x 450 kg x 12.25 Dkr :	165
Slaughtered after calving	0.76 x 510 kg x 11.28 Dkr :	4,372	0.19 x 520 kg x 11.28 Dkr :	1,114
Cows entering second lactation			0.77 x 8,744 Dkr :	6,733
Calves (90% surviving)	0.68 x 1,400 Dkr :	952	0.86 x 1,400 Dkr :	1,204
Milk yield (4%)	1254 kg x 2.30 Dkr :	2,884	4470 kg x 2.30 Dkr :	10,280
Total		**9,452**		**19.498**
Expenses				
Female calf	:	1,600	:	1,600
Feed consumed	:	6,391	:	10,701
Veterinary, etc.	:	536	:	277
Materials	:	260	:	484
Total		**8,787**		**13,062**
Returns		**665**		**6,436**
Labour, invest. man-hours		43		73
Loss per infected pregnant heifer		5,771 Dkr		

Expenses per animal comprised costs of the newborn female calf, total feed consumption, expenses in association with the disease outbreak, i.e. 336 Dkr (see above) plus additional veterinary medical care of 200 Dkr. making a total of 536 Dkr. Further management costs were 260 Dkr. It appears that at the termination of first lactation, the calculated excess of income over expenditure amounted to 665 Dkr. for the affected animal and 6,436 Dkr. for the non-affected, the difference, i.e. loss, per animal being 5,771 Dkr. (5,800 Dkr.).

This loss is not corrected for difference in labour investment, *i.e.* 43 man-hours per affected animal and 73 man-hours per non-affected, because incidence and practical consequences of outbreaks cannot be predicted and taken into account in the management planning.

Non-pregnant heifers

At the time of the acute outbreak the average age of the 34 non-pregnant heifers was 618 days but the variation was high (437-919 days). The calculated average weight was 350 kg. Out of the affected animals 0,3% died from acute illness. The remaining animals were all slaughtered after treatment and restorement, and insemination was not attempted. The time interval until slaughter varied greatly. On average it was 4 months, which allowed an (estimated) average gain of approximately 50 kg per animal. Calculation of the economical loss per animal was made as described for pregnant heifers above (Table 1). It constituted 1,964 Dkr. (2,000 Dkr.) per affected animal and the labour investment was 20 man-hours and 27 man-hours for the summer mastitis infected and the non-infected heifer respectively. The total loss per animal was not corrected for this labour difference.

The marked difference in loss between the summer mastitis infected pregnant and non-pregnant heifers may, in part, be seen in the light of differences in age and weight at the time of the attack, but even more in the partial failure of the pregnant heifer to contribute to the first lactation and the complete dismissal of the heifer from the dairy herd before the second lactation period. Losses in both pregnant and non-pregnant heifers are certainly highly related to the genetical value of a given herd. The ongoing genetically determined increase of performance is believed to be diminished by the early removal of recruitment stock, but the actual economical impact of this phenomenon is difficult to define.

Estimated benefits from preventive measures in relation to incidence rates and category of heifers

Table 2 illustrates estimated losses, at different incidence rates, per 100 head of pregnant and non-pregnant heifers respectively. The losses listed in the table have been worked out on the basis of the calculated average loss per animal described above. We operate with two hypothetical preventive strategies: One which may reduce the incidence by 75% and which may cost 3,000 Dkr. per 100 animals (*e.g.* ear-tags), and one which ensures complete (100%) prevention, *e.g.* by housing animals in July and August, a tradition which an increasing number of farmers tend to follow. This latter practice, involving extra stable-feeding, management etc. will cost 26,000 Dkr. per 100 pregnant heifers and 17,500 Dkr. per 100 non-pregnant heifers. It will be seen that the "cheap" strategy, reducing expected incidence by 75%, is superior in terms of "returns" when applied to non-pregnant heifers even having high expected incidences and also when applied to pregnant heifers with expected low or moderate incidences. Only in pregnant heifers at high risk was housing economically slightly superior. However, in intensive herds with high genetical progress, housing would possibly be superior even at lower incidence rates.

TABLE 2.   Benefits per 100 animals from two preventive measures in relation to various (expected) incidence rates in pregnant and non-pregnant heifers

Incidence rate % (expected)	Losses (Dkr) without prevention	"Returns" (Dkr) from prevention	
		75%	100%
Pregnant			
20	115,000	83,000	89,000
10	58,000	40,500	32,000
5	29,000	19,000	3,000
Non-pregnant			
20	39,000	26,000	21,500
10	19,500	12,000	2,000
5	10,000	4,500	− 7,500

There is certainly a tremendous need for development of highly protective measures which would allow pregnant heifers to graze at negligable risk throughout the season.

SUMMER MASTITIS IN BELGIUM
GEOGRAPHICAL DISTRIBUTION AND ECONOMIC LOSS

G. Bertels

Verbond voor dierziektenbestrijding van Limburg,
Opsporingscentrum, Wetserstraat 14,
B 3820 — Alken, Belgium.

ABSTRACT

After inventarisation of the summer mastitis regions in Belgium, we counted the number of cattle in these regions and also the number of calves and heifers. About 30% of these summer mastitis regions had a sandy soil and 70% a loam soil. There was a remarkably good correlation between the wooded area of Belgium and the summer mastitis areas. Loss per case was estimated at 444 E.C.U. for pure milk types, 222 E.C.U. for mixed types and 100 E.C.U. for meat types. Given an incidence of 2% summer mastitis in young cattle we calculated for Belgium a loss of 800,000 E.C.U. on 150,000 milking type animals, 523,000 E.C.U. on 197,000 mixed type animals and 668,000 E.C.U. on 789,000 meat type animals. The same calculation was done for a 6% summer mastitis incidence. The total loss in Belgium amounts to 5,770,000 E.C.U. for 6% summer mastitis and 2,000,000 E.C.U. for 2% summer mastitis. Finally, we estimated the maximum costs for summer mastitis prevention with a 2% incidence. Per animal, this was 8.90 E.C.U., 4.40 E.C.U., and 2.00 E.C.U. for milk-, mixed-, and meat types respectively.

INTRODUCTION

In this study an attempt was made to make an inventarisation of the summer mastitis areas, the number of animals and economic loss in Belgium. Detailed information on this subject was lacking.

ECONOMIC LOSS PER CASE

The first step was to make an estimation of the economic loss per case of summer mastitis for the different races (Table 1). To do this we divided the cattle into 3 groups: pure milking types (Friesian, Holstein), mixed types (Red-White, Black-White, etc.) and meat types (mainly White-Blue Belgian).

In meat races there is only a loss in fattening, milk is of little importance. Conclusion: there are great differences in economical loss from summer mastitis between the different groups.

SUMMER MASTITIS AREAS IN BELGIUM

A distribution of summer mastitis areas in Belgium was made based on questionaires distributed by the Veterinary Health Service to local practising veterinarians. The results are summarised in Fig. 1.

TABLE 1.   Loss estimates for the three groups of cattle in Belgium in E.C.U.

	Milk	Mixed	Meat
Commercial value pregnant heifer	1,000	1,000	
Loss in milk yield -10%	106	106	
Cost for fattening		115	100
Value of calf	107	222	
Slaughter value	555	777	
Loss	444 E.C.U.	222 E.C.U.	100 E.C.U.

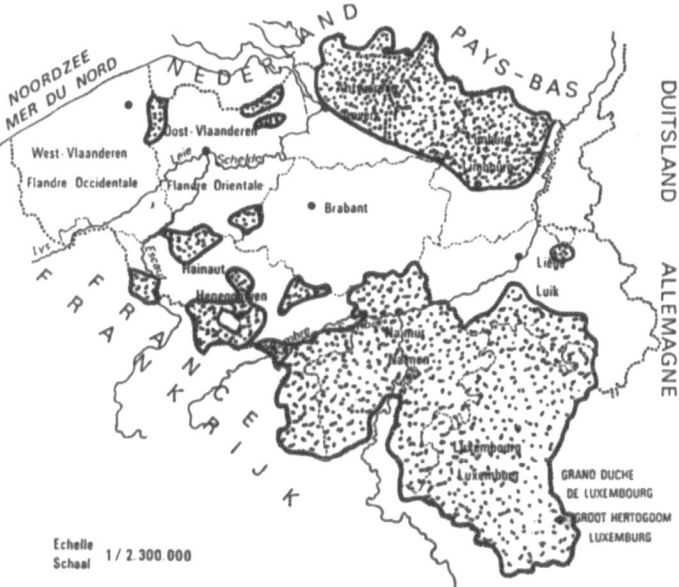

Fig. 1. Areas of Belgium having a known history of summer mastitis.

In the literature, summer mastitis has been associated with areas having sandy soils. This is certainly the case for the Belgian province of Limburg. We also attempted to find this association in the other summer mastitis regions (see Fig. 2) but found that only 30% of all these areas had sandy soil whereas 70% had a loamy soil.

A much better correlation was found between wooded regions and the summer mastitis areas of Belgium (see Fig. 3).

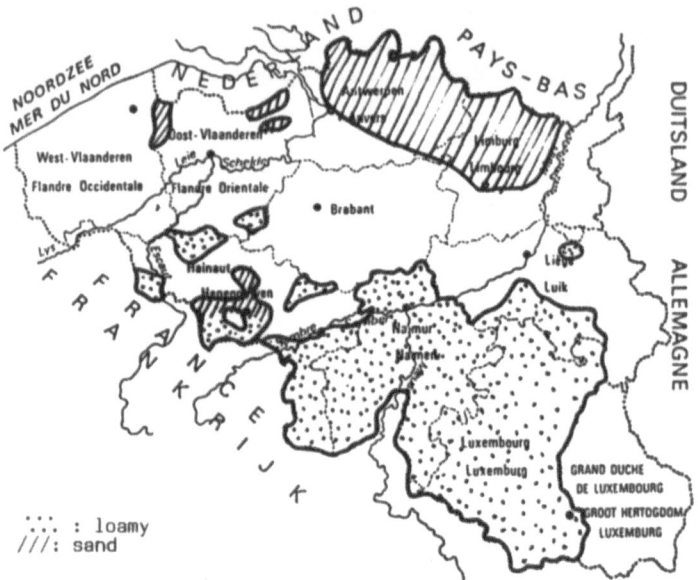

Fig. 2. The association between soil type and summer mastitis areas in Belgium.

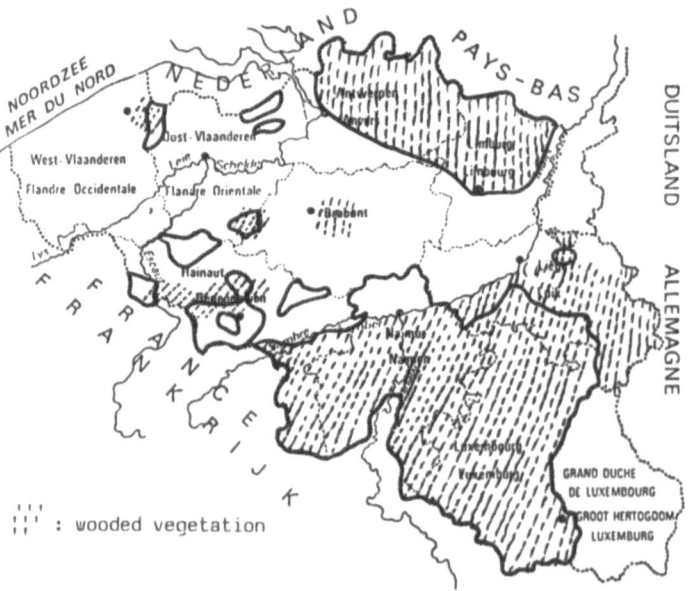

Fig. 3. Map of Belgium showing regions with wooded vegetation (hatched area) and known summer mastitis areas (bold outline).

In conclusion, as far as Belgium is concerned, a wooded vegetation is a more important factor than the soil type.

NUMBER OF CATTLE AND THE ECONOMIC LOSS

There are 3 million cattle in Belgium. The number of cattle in the summer mastitis areas may be estimated from the annual counting of cattle. The number of animals at risk, that is, calves and heifers, were estimated from the totals in the different groups at about 60% for milk and mixed types and 42% for meat types. These figures were then used to determine the losses that would occur with summer mastitis incidences of 6% and 2%. These data are given in Table 2.

TABLE 2.   Data used to estimate the loss with a 6% and 2% incidence of summer mastitis in the different suspected areas in Belgium.

	Group	Limberg	Antwerp	E.Flanders	Henegouwen	Namen	Luik	Luxemberg	Total
Total	milk	12,449	120,000	17,588	—	—	—	—	150,000
numbers	mixed	12,449	120,000	35,176	21,330	—	8,000	—	197,000
animals	meat	—	—	17,588	181,902	250,000	32,000	307,729	789,000
Number	milk	7,469	72,000	10,552	—	—	—	—	90,000
calves	mixed	7,469	72,000	21,105	12,789	—	4,800	—	118,000
+ heifers	meat	—	—	7,387	76,398	105,000	13,440	131,874	334,000
No. cases	milk	448	4,320	633	—	—	—	—	4,950
6%	mixed	448	4,320	1,266	767	—	288	—	7,090
	meat	—	—	443	4,583	6,300	806	7,912	20,000
2%	milk	149	1,440	211	—	—	—	—	1,800
	mixed	149	1,440	422	255	—	96	—	2,360
	meat	—	—	147	1,527	2,100	268	2,637	6,680
Economic	milk	198,984	1,918,080	281,105	—	—	—	—	2,200,000
loss in ECU	mixed	99,456	959,040	281,052	170,469	—	—	—	1,570,000
6%	meat	—	—	44,300	458,393	630,000	80,600	791,200	2,000,000
2%	milk	66,324	639,360	93,701	—	—	—	—	800,000
	mixed	33,078	959,040	93,706	56,823	—	21,312	—	523,000
	meat	—	—	14,774	152,798	210,000	26,800	263,700	668,000

As far as Belgium is concerned the loss with a total of 1,136,000 animals at risk in suspected areas comes to 5,770,000 E.C.U. when the incidence is 6% and 2,000,000 E.C.U. when this is 2%.

MAXIMUM COSTS FOR PREVENTION

The above given losses were also used to determine the maximum cost per animal that the farmer may spend on summer mastitis prevention. The formula used was

$$\frac{\text{N. potential mastitis cases X loss per individual within that group}}{\text{total N. animals at risk within that group}}$$

With a 6% summer mastitis incidence, the estimated amounts that may be spent are 24.4, 13.3, and 6.0 E.C.U. for milk, mixed and meat types respectively. When the incidence is 2% these amounts will be 8.9, 4.4 and 2.0 E.C.U's respectively.

REFERENCES

Douna, M.L. 1972. LEI publication 3.33.

Kronborg, D., Morup, A., Hansen, J.W., Nansen, P., Foldager, J. and Willeberg, P. 1985. En epidemiologisk undersogelse af sommermastitis hos kvier, samt en vurdering af forebyggende princippers effekt. In: Report on summer mastitis to the Danish Veterinary and Agricultural Research Council, Chapter 11.

Madsen, M., Nielsen, S. Achim and Nansen, P. 1986. Sommermastitis. Praesentation af et 4-årigt forskningsprojekt II. Transmission, epidemiologi, immunologi og forebyggelse. Dansk Vet. Tidsskr., **69**, 533-543.

Sorensen, G.H. 1979. Sommermastitis. Thesis. Carl Fr. Mortensen A/S, Kobenhavn.

Oestergaard, V. 1983a. Optimale foderrationer til malkekoen under forskellige forudsaetninger. I. "Optimale foderrationer till malkekoen". 551. beretning fra Statens Husdyrbrugsforsog. Kobenhavn. 18.1-18.49.

Oestergaard, V. 1983b. Faktor- og produktpriser i kvaegbedriften 1982/83. 552. beretning fra Statens Husdyrbrugsforsog. Kobenhavn. 15-17.

Tolle, A. and Reichmuth, J. 1985. Summer mastitis. Kiel. Milch. Forschung., **37** (4), 575-584.

DISCUSSION

In the discussion following the session a general concensus of opinion was reached with regard to the majority of econ-ergonomic models formulated to estimate the cost of summer mastitis in the different member countries of the EEC. It was considered possible that assessments are, on the whole, underestimates of the real cost and that three problem areas exist which contribute to this error.

1. It was pointed out that very few models incorporate costings for labour differences deriving from care of summer mastitic animals as compared to healthy animals. In strict economic terms this aspect of cost should be incorporated *e.g.* as an hourly rate. In the discussion that followed it emerged that one of the reasons why these forms of calculation cannot be done is that the very variable incidence of summer mastitis from year to year makes it imposible to predict labour requirements. Moreover, the specific situation of the farmer varies greatly between individuals, *i.e.* distance from farm buildings, labour requirement for harvesting which coincides with the peak in summer mastitis incidence *etc.*

2. The second problem area is provided by a rather intangable cost for the farmer — the worry due to the unpredictability of the disease. This appears to be an important factor when mixed farms are the rule and the farmer spends most of the time harvesting and works from early morning until late at night exactly at the peak of the summer mastitis season. Consequently, it is very troublesome to have to go and handle diseased animals. Worry is one of the main reasons underlying the currently growing practice of housing animals in Denmark to ensure being on the safe side despite the extra and often unnecessary costs involved.

The development of an effective warning system would be of great value in reducing costs in both of the above areas.

3. The final point raised in the discussion related to the costs of research into summer mastitis. Up until now this has been funded at the national level, usually in precipitous spurts as response to particularly severe outbreaks of summer mastitis. As a consequence costs vary and are somewhat correlated with the, as yet, unpredicable incidence of the disease. The session was concluded by discussing the impact of workshops on the relative costs and benefits of research. It was ratified that these were highly profitable in at least two ways. Firstly, exchange of information at an early stage is certain to reduce research costs at the national level. Secondly, they result in invaluable contacts with relevent research programs between individual laboratories and countries. Moreover, it was pointed out that some areas within the very complex problem of summer mastitis are, experimentally, extremely expensive to run at the size and/or in the circumstances required to achieve a solution, *e.g.* experimental infections, fly studies in relation to large variation in incidence *etc.* At the national level these are beyond the resources of individual research councils but co-operation and

coordinated division of labour at the C.E.C. or international level would present an effective method of cost reduction in this type of expensive research.

7. CONCLUSIONS AND RECOMMENDATIONS

CONCLUSIONS AND RECOMMENDATIONS

INTRODUCTION

Farmers and their agricultural and veterinary advisors have for many years recognized a syndrome/condition described as "summer mastitis", "heifer mastitis", "―――".

The syndrome is confined to non-lactating pastured cattle during the summer months. Since the early seventies this syndrome has created increasing concern among farmers' organizations and agricultural economists. It is predominantly localized in the north-western European maritime region. There is a marked variation in incidence from year to year and from locality to locality but mathematical epidemiological assessment is lacking. The most severe illness with the most serious prognosis is due to a combination of certain anaerobes and *C. pyogenes*. A similar combination of bacteria is also found at other times of the year with same seriousness but lower incidence.

EPIDEMIOLOGY

Enzootic mastitis in non-lactating cattle is restricted to the western maritime region of Europe in the summer and autumn although a significant number of cases occur in spring in some areas. The epidemiology with respect to annual incidence, seasonal pattern, age of cattle, quarter of the udder infected and incidence of different breeds is well documented.

A priority in understanding the disease better should be mathematical modelling of the epidemiology augmented by investigation of the poorly understood effects of breeding strategy and pregnancy. Information on similar infections known from other geographical areas, throughout the year and in lactating cattle will also be useful as these may be of increasing importance.

BACTERIOLOGY

The papers presented within this session generally agreed upon the complex bacterial background of the disease. Bacteriological investigations of summer mastitis secretions have revealed the presence of a complex of micro-aerophilic and obligate anaerobic bacteria of which the most frequently recovered species are *Corynebacterium* (s. *Actinomyces*) *pyogenes*, *Peptococcus indolicus*, the Stuart-Schwann (s. "micro-aerophilic") coccus, *Fusobacterium necrophorum*, *Bacteroides melaninogenicus* and *Streptococcus dysgalactiae*.

At least two of these species are required to reproduce the clinical disease experimentally, but the knowledge available with regard to bacterial interactions, synergistic effects, *etc.* within this very complex microbial ecosystem is presently limited, and should thus be thoroughly investigated.

An impressive spectrum of virulence factors has been demonstrated within the involved bacterial species, some of which are important in the establishment of the infection (*e.g.* pili, adhesion factors), some in the evasion of the host immune response (*e.g.* leucocidin, Ig-proteases) and some responsible for the tissue destruction (*e.g.* hemolysin, necrotoxins). Further research work with regard to the proper biochemical characterization and the significance of these virulence factors is very much required and strongly recommended.

AETIOLOGY / PATHOGENESIS

Experiments show that intramammary inoculation with monocultures of the batches of the bacteria isolated from field cases of summer mastitis do not reliably reproduce the disease.

Simultaneous or sequential challenge with *Corynebacterium pyogenes* and *Peptococcus indolicus* is effective in causing summer mastitis as are some other combinations involving obligate anaerobic bacteria.

The mechanisms of natural infection, the dynamics of the infection process and the interactions among the bacteria and with the host which lead to disease are not understood. Furthermore, little research is in progress with respect to the nature of the host's immunological response to disease although this is relevant to pathogenesis.

Research is recommended in the following areas:

1. The interactions between the bacteria implicated in summer mastitis with special emphasis on growth conditions, microbial physiology and the elaboration of colonisation, toxic and anti-host factors.
2. The physiological and immunological factors responsible for the particular susceptibility of the non-lactating mammary gland to summer mastitis require eludication.

TRANSMISSION OF THE DISEASE

Literature studies show that two hypotheses have been proposed to explain summer mastitis:

a) Endogenous infection plus increased stress in summer possibly from flies.
b) Vector transmission via cattle visiting Diptera probably *Hydrotaea irritans.*

More information is required in the following areas:

1. Very little is known regarding the endogenous hypothesis — at the moment it remains an observation. More work is necessary in this area, particularly with respect to whether flies are also involved in distributing bacteria which are present as sub-clinical infections in cattle and to investigate the role of the fly as a potential stressor.
2. Concentration is currently placed on the role of *H. irritans* as the vector of summer mastitis. Although this is valid given the information available at the moment it is also necessary to retain an open mind and not ignore other potential vectors and also interactions between biting and sucking insects.
3. The only remaining obstacle weakening the vector transmission hypothesis via *H. irritans*

is the inability to repeat the early transmission experiments. More attention has to be paid to this, particularly by integrating all the information that is available to generate effective models that describe the optimal parameters necessary for transmission.

PREVENTION AND THERAPY

It is realized that the control of summer mastitis needs optimalization.

With regard to prevention there is evidence that the present application of insecticides is not effective enough and, in the long run, might lead to undesirable side-effects (resistance in insect populations, "environmental" problems). An alternative preventive method could be to manipulate the fly population by using, for example, optimal fly traps. These could also function in an early warning system.

It is advised to continue basic research with regard to the aetiology and pathogenesis of the disease and evaluate the perspective resulting from recent developments in the field of molecular biology aiming at immunization.

In the field of therapy more insight is needed into the relation between clinical picture, the bacteriology of the disease and the effect of treatment.

ECONOMICS AND ERGONOMICS

Considering the economic and ergonomic implications of summer mastitis from the aspect of selecting the manner of prevention appropriate for an individual situation an urgent need is felt to provide dairy farmers in areas at risk with comparative information on all the methods of prevention and their efficacy to allow them a better decision base.

It is critical that more emphasis is given to developing an early warning system, as prediction of incidence would allow a more efficient allocation of cost factors for prevention.

The development of efficient prevention is dependent on long term research. This is currently funded at the national level. Short Community and other international workshops can help to reduce these costs by encouraging exchange of information at an early stage. Some areas within the very complex problem of summer mastitis are, experimentally, extremely expensive to run at the size and/or in the circumstances required to achieve a solution, *e.g.* experimental infections, fly studies in relation to large variation in incidence *etc.* At the national level these are beyond the resources of individual research councils. It is recommended that encouragement of co-operation and coordinated division of labour at an international level might implement an effective method in improving research progress.

LIST OF PARTICIPANTS

Dr. G. Bertels, Provinciaal Opsporingscentrum, Wetserstraat 14, B—3820 Alken, Belgium.

Dr. A.E.J.M. van den Bogaard, Dienst Centrale Proefdiervoorziening, R.U. Limburg, Postbus 616, 6200 MD Maastricht, The Netherlands.

Dr. A.J. Bramley, Institute for Research on Animal Diseases, Compton, Berkshire, RG16 ONN, U.K.

Dr. J. Chirico, Dept. of Parasitology, National Veterinary Institute, Box 7073, S—750 07 Uppsala, Sweden.

Dr. J. Connell, Commission of the European Communities, 200 Rue de la Loi, 1049 Brussels, Belgium.

Dr. R. De Deken, Instituut v. Tropische Geneeskunde "Prins Leopold", Nationalestraat 155, B—2000 Antwerp, Belgium.

Dr. P. Fagiolo, Istituto Zooprofilattico Sperimentale del Lazio e della Toscana, Via Appia Roma, Capannelle, Italy.

Dr. J.E. Hillerton, Institute for Research on Animal Diseases, Compton, Berkshire, RG16 ONN, U.K.

Prof. O. Holmberg, National Veterinary Institute, Box 7073, S—750 07 Uppsala, Sweden.

Dr. J.B. Jespersen, Danish Pest Infestation Laboratory, Skovbrynet 14, DK—2800 Lyngby, Denmark.

Dr. P. Jonsson, National Veterinary Institute, Box 7073, S—750 07 Uppsala, Sweden.

Prof. A. Liebisch, Institut für Parasitologie, Tierärtztlichen Hochschule, Bunteweg 17, D—3000, Hannover 71, F.R.G.

Dr. M. Madsen, Royal Veterinary and Agricultural University, Institute of Hygiene and Microbiology, 13 Bülowsvej, DK—1870 Copenhagen V, Denmark.

Dr. W. Meaney, The Agricultural Institute, Moorepark Research Centre, Fermoy, Country Cork, Ireland.

Prof. P. Nansen, Royal Veterinary and Agricultural University, Institute of Hygiene and Microbiology, 13 Bülowsvej, DK—1870 Copenhagen V, Denmark.

Dr. S.A. Nielsen, Roskilde University Center, Institute of Biology and Chemistry, Marbjergvej 45, P.O. Box 260, DK—4000, Roskilde, Denmark.

Dr. S.-O. Olsson, Association for Swedish Livestock Breeding and Production, S—631 84 Eskilstuna, Sweden.

Dr. H.J. Over, Dept. Parasitology, Central Veterinary Institute, Postbus 65, 8200 AB Lelystad, The Netherlands.

Dr. B. Overgaard Nielsen, Institute of Zoology and Zoophysiology, Zoological Laboratory, Universitetsparken, Build. 135, DK—8000 Aarhus C, Denmark.

Dr. J. Reichmuth, Institut für Hygiene, Bundesanstalt für Milchforschung, Herman—Weigmann—Strasse 1, Postfach 6069 D—2300, Kiel 14, F.R.G.

Dr. J.M.F. Saes, Gezondheidsdienst v. Dieren Prov. Limburg, Postbus 3100, 6093 ZJ Heythuysen, The Netherlands.

Dr. **J.W. Seinhorst**, Proefstation v.d. Rundveehouderij, Runderweg 6, 8219 PK Lelystad, The Netherlands.

Dr. **J. Sol**, Gezondheidsdienst v. Dieren Prov. Overijssel, Postbus 13, 8000 AA Zwolle, The Netherlands.

Dr. **G. Thomas**, Dept. Parasitology, Central Veterinary Institute, Postbus 65, 8200 AB Lelystad, The Netherlands.

Prof. **P. Tsakalof**, Dept. of Obstetrics and A.I., Veterinary School, Aristotelian University of Thessaloniki, 11 Stavrou Voutryra St., Thessaloniki, Greece.

Dr. **U. Vecht**, Dept. Bacteriology, Central Veterinary Institute, Postbus 65, 8200 AB Lelystad, The Netherlands.

Dr. **G. de Vries**, Stichting Gezondheidszorg v. Dieren, Prinsevinkenpark 24, 2585 HL 's-Gravenhage, The Netherlands.

Dr. **C.A. Watson**, MAFF, Veterinary Investigation Centre, Langford House, Langford, Bristol BSi8 7DX, U.K.

Dr. **A. Zecconi**, Facolta di medicina Veterinaria Di Milano, Istituto di malattie infecttive, Via Celoria 10, 20133 Milano, Italy.

ASSOCIATE PARTICIPANTS

Mr. **M.J. van den Berg**, Dept. Animal Physiology, University of Groningen, Postbus 14, 9750 AA Haren, The Netherlands.

Mr. **L. Beukeboom**, Dept. Genetics, University of Groningen, Kerklaan 30, 9751 NN Haren, The Netherlands.

Mr. **J.A.J. Breeuwer**, Dept. Animal Physiology, University of Groningen, Postbus 14, 9750 AA Haren, The Netherlands.

Prof. **H.J. Breukink**, Faculty of Veterinary Medicine, Yalelaan 16, 3584 CM Utrecht, The Netherlands.

Mr. **J.N. van der Linden**, Dept. Parasitology, Central Veterinary Institute, Postbus 65, 8200 AB Lelystad, The Netherlands.

Mr. **H.J. Prijs**, Dept. Parasitology, Central Veterinary Institute, Postbus 65, 8200 AB Lelystad, The Netherlands.

Miss **E.R.M. Verheijen**, Dept. Bacteriology, Central Veterinary Institute, Postbus 65, 8200 AB Lelystad, The Netherlands.

Mr. **H.J. Wisselink**, Dept. Bacteriology, Central Veterinary Institute, Postbus 65, 8200 AB Lelystad, The Netherlands.